The Thinking Person's Guide To Fitness

The Thinking Person's Guide To Fitness

What THEY don't tell you about
looking and feeling great!

By Jake Nash

Dedicated to my family:
My mother and sister without whom I couldn't
have made it here and my father for
everything.

Special Thanks to:
Cynthia Barzyk Sullivan
and
Phil Petersen
Without whom this book
would be a comical mess.

Table of Contents

Part I - The Philosophy of Fitness

"It is dangerous to be right in matters on which the established authorities are wrong." Voltaire

If you think there's a shortcut to fitness, this book is not for you. If you don't want to understand what you're doing in the gym, and just want a book that tells you what to do and not why, then this book is not for you. If you enjoy hanging out in the gym, and don't have anything better to do with your time, then this book is not for you. If you only trust the exercise recommendations of the "authorities" in our government and other stodgy institutions, then this book is not for you. If you are easily offended by politically incorrect thoughts, facts or theories, then it is also not for you.

However, if you are intelligent and a free thinker, this book IS for you. If you want to optimize your fitness program, this book IS for you. If you've long ago learned that the best way to be successful in ANY area of your life is to have at least a basic understanding of that subject, and you want to understand how your body works without getting a degree in exercise science...this book IS for you. If you're not afraid to think outside the box, and if you'd like to learn from someone who is BOTH technically educated and has the experience of working with hundreds of people just like you, THEN THIS BOOK IS FOR YOU!

This is not "Fitness for Dummies". Nor is it one of many other books on the shelves that will give you a one-size-fits-all solution to your fitness needs, regardless of your goals or individual situation. Yes, you can make progress with the fitness plans outlined in any of these other books, but it will not be optimum progress. It will take you longer to reach your goals, and you will have to spend more time in the gym than if you had a program customized to you and your goals.

1

How do you get a custom program? Well, you have two options: You can educate yourself, or you can hire an expert.

You might say "I don't want to have to become a fitness expert, I'd rather just hire a trainer." That's a great idea, but how do you know who to hire? In my time in the industry, I have interviewed at least 300 trainers for positions at my studios (probably closer to 500). From my experience, 80% of them are worthless, and perhaps 5% truly know what they are doing. The sad fact is, among hard core fitness buffs, personal trainers are somewhat of a joke, an amusing part of any gym. Most of us cringe as we watch these less than knowledgeable trainers take their clients through some pretty useless workouts.

So how will you find the 5% that can really help you, or how do you teach yourself enough about fitness that you can do it yourself? That's the purpose of this book. It's not intended to be a "how to" book on getting in shape. Nor is it the be-all-end-all book of knowledge on health and fitness. You won't find tons of exercise descriptions or recipes that you can find in many other sources, although I will give you references to the good places to find those.

What you will find is a comprehensive list of all the mistakes and misunderstandings that I see on a day-to-day basis with my clients. These clients are most often successful, educated, intelligent people, who, for one or many of the reasons listed in Chapter 1 have opinions or beliefs about exercise and diet that are leading them to waste their time, all the while not getting the results they desire.

I will not waste your time repeating things you've seen a hundred times before, unless I truly feel it's an issue that still needs to be addressed. Not all of my clients suffer from all of these errors, but each error is common enough that no matter how commonly available the information is, it obviously needs to be repeated.

As such, if you're just looking for someone to tell you what to do and mindlessly how to do it, this is not the book for you.

This is written for the reader who wants to understand why they do what they do and knows that a one-size-fits-all fitness program is not for them.

The person who finds this book useful is the person who values not only their fitness, but also their time. They are tired of being lied to, and tired of programs that never work as well as advertised. They are willing to put a little time into learning about the basics so that they can then figure out what works for them.

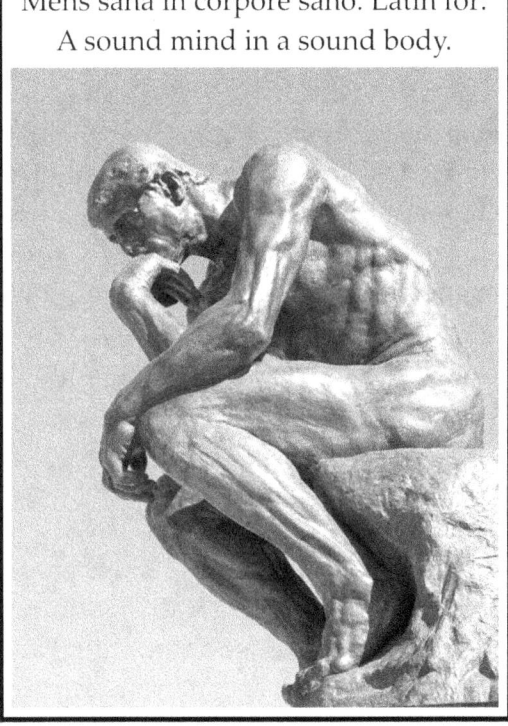

Mens sana in corpore sano. Latin for: A sound mind in a sound body.

Yes, there are other books out there that will educate you instead of just giving you a program, but most of them assume you are already in the industry. They are written for athletes, trainers, bodybuilders, fitness models, etc. This book bridges the gap. Once you understand the material presented here, you'll be able to pick up those books, most of which are written on specific topics, and understand what they are talking about.

But be warned…I don't pull any punches! This material is straight up and blunt. If you're the politically correct, sensitive type, this book may not be for you.

Ok, let's get started!!

Chapter 1 – Intro - Don't Die of a Misprint

Be careful about reading health books. You may die of a misprint. - Mark Twain

Yes, that's quite a way to start out a health and fitness book, but what Mark Twain knew over a hundred years ago is as true today as it was then. Fact is, most of us have gotten used to being lied to and deceived when it comes to our health and fitness. It's almost like it's just part of the game: useless gadgets and gimmicks, fads, and new exercise programs with fancy names, and new diets, each one purporting to allow us to lose weight while we eat everything in sight and don't exercise.

If you're not fed up with it by now, you're lucky. You either haven't been struggling with a fitness goal or you're really patient.

I don't want to start off by disparaging other very competent people, but if you've been paying attention, you've probably figured out that most of the people giving you advice are not qualified to be giving you advice. Your personal physician may be great at diagnosing disease, but probably had less than a single class on nutrition, and probably no education at all on exercise. The "registered dietician" giving you advice on the proper way to eat had a curriculum entirely based on clinical nutrition, or how diseased people should be fed in a hospital, not how to eat to look good in a bathing suit. Your personal trainer probably had a weekend long course in exercise, and may not even have a basic fundamental understanding of the scientific theory behind the exercises they select for you. Many of the "experts" you see on TV are no more than pretty faces and hot bodies and in reality have never even used the device or diet they are selling. How about your super "buff" friend? Chances are he has some pretty great genetics, or even some "pharmaceutical assistance." He'd probably look great no matter what he did. Let's face it, unless you are a professional athlete, the fitness advice you are getting is at best woefully lacking.

It's not their fault. All the professionals giving you fitness advice were never really educated in how it all works. Why would they even bother to get that education? Our system is just not set up to value that kind of knowledge. Even the personal trainer will not end up any more successful if they pursue a higher knowledge level. They will make far more money from their personality or whatever the latest fitness gadget or gimmick may be.

That's where this book comes in. I've helped close to a thousand real people in the real world achieve their fitness goals. I've always prided myself on NOT using gadgets and gimmicks, NOT relying on fads with fancy names to attract clients, and ALWAYS telling it like it is.

Much of the information in this book is available elsewhere. Some of it you may find in the more up-to-date fitness magazines and web sites (some are actually very good if you bother to find and read them), but a lot of it you won't find anywhere outside research reports and highly specialized publications. Some of it is certainly very specific to my own methods, and if you find it elsewhere it just proves the old adage that there are very few actual original ideas in the world.

Reasons Fitness Errors are so Prevalent

I already opened this section by telling you that you may be listening to the wrong people when it comes to fitness advice. If you're already satisfied that the fitness advice you've been getting is not generally accurate, you can skip to the next section.

There are some very significant problems with health and fitness research. First, it is very hard to generate good data as it relates to the human body. The human body is VERY complex. Pharmaceutical companies spend many millions of dollars to study each and every interaction and effect of every drug they manufacture, and sometimes they still miss the mark. However, studies on health and fitness are generally done for graduate level university studies that, at best, are underfunded, and usually woefully lacking in proper experimental design, if for no other reason than just lack of study participants. There are often 10-20 participants in studies that should be run on 50-100 or more.

The VAST majority of health and fitness studies are done on 18-20 year old college freshmen. If you can remember that time in your life, you're probably thinking the same thing I do: their lifestyles, eating habits, recovery ability, and hormonal levels, among many other factors, are all very unrepresentative of your average overworked 38 year old mother of 3 and/or corporate executive.

The data generated, is usually very restricted in the conclusions that can be drawn from it. However, as in mainstream media, that doesn't stop the researchers and health and fitness publications from sometimes overreaching.

I was an engineer in a laboratory for many years. In that time I ran more studies than I can remember. Many of them were inconclusive. That is, you really couldn't draw any conclusions one way or another, or you could draw conclusions, but they were either counter to conventional wisdom, or raised more questions than they answered.

That's how science works. Unfortunately, most bosses (or professors) want answers, right or wrong. When someone gives you money to run a test, and you come back with "inconclusive" as the result, there's a tremendous amount of pressure to "make up" an answer. Since the human body is so complex, bad conclusions from inconclusive data seem to be more common than not.

There's also the problem of the whole second hand news phenomenon. When you read a health article in a magazine or online, it's most often written by a reporter who is putting their own spin on the researcher's results. Sometimes, an erroneous spin.

I saw this many times during my years in the laboratory, and I became very good at "reading between the lines" to figure out what a study really said. Have you heard the saying "Statistics don't lie but liars use statistics"? Well there's an even better one as it applies to this topic. I hope the wording doesn't offend anyone, but the applicability here is so strong that I can't help using it: "according to statistics, the average American has one ball and one breast." Have you ever met such an individual?

I'll give you an example that came up as I was writing this. In a study I saw quoted a lot, researchers studied the forces on your spine and surrounding muscles under various seated positions. What they found was that the forces were higher when seated straight up than when the individual leaned back in a reclined position.

The conclusion that I saw reported four times was that we should all start leaning back while we're seated. Really? Did the study actually run for many years and measure back problems in people who sat up straight versus those who reclined? No, of course they didn't. Instead, the researchers and reporters drew conclusions with insufficient data.

You see, as anyone who is well researched in lower back disorders knows, continual loading of the lower back musculature is REQUIRED for optimum back health. It's why astronauts have to be very careful to exercise while in space, and even so will experience muscular atrophy that they must recover from once they return to earth. It's also the reason why any modern surgeon will have a back surgery patient out of bed and walking mere days after the surgery.

Lower back health is not about avoiding the use of these core muscles, it's about constantly exercising them with forces that are large enough to keep them strong and healthy, but low enough to not cause damage. Standing or sitting with proper straight posture does load your spine to some small degree (well below any level that could cause damage), but also requires your muscles to engage in a continuous workout in order to maintain the upright posture (hence why we slump when we get lazy or tired).

The reports did correctly report that slouching over in your chair is not good because it not only places higher loads on your spine, but it relaxes all of the surrounding musculature. The study generated correct data, however the conclusions everyone is generating are simply incorrect. You'll learn more about back health later, but I thought this example would be good up front because it is such a simple yet significant example of how bad interpretation of studies in this industry can point us in such a dangerously wrong direction.

Watch just about anyone sitting at the computer, dinner table, etc., and chances are they look like the photo on the left. Years of sitting like this can be just as destructive to your spine as a much more dramatic accident. Sitting like the right picture will not hurt your spine (contrary to the badly reported research).

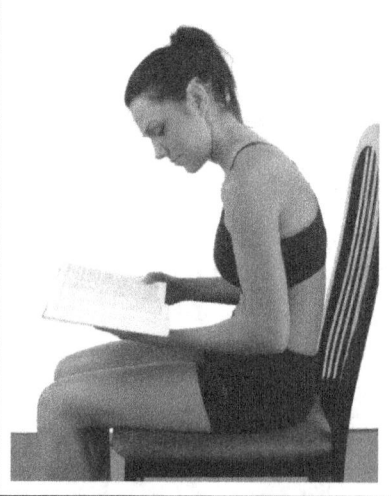 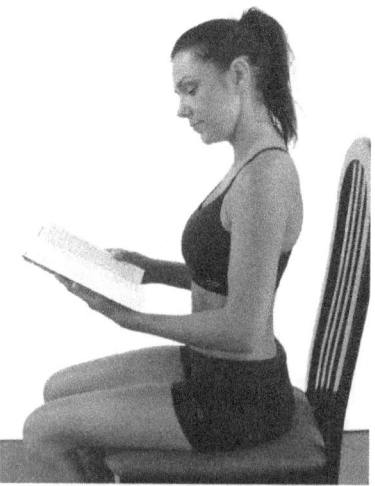

You've seen the same thing happen throughout the health and fitness world: First eggs were good for you, then they were not, now they're a good, healthy food again. The researchers didn't necessarily make the mistakes generating the data, but whoever drew the conclusions went further than the data allowed.

To make matters worse, everything seems to change from year to year. The fact is, we know very little about how the human body works. Even modern medicine is just a series of best guesses. We've yet to scratch the surface of the vast complexity that is the human body.

Although we're not going to talk about treating disease in this book, there are similarities as they apply to the human body. Until very recently, disease was treated in a very general fashion: If you had a certain disease, you were given a specific medication or surgery. Sometimes, it worked and sometimes it didn't, but no one ever knew why. Your doctor never said, "Well you're of Scandinavian decent, and we know this treatment doesn't seem to work well on Scandinavians, so we'll try something else". The standard treatment either worked or it didn't.

Very recently, medical researchers have discovered that not only can a disease itself vary from person to person, but the persons very own DNA can actually affect and determine what treatment will work and what won't work. The latest cancer treatments being developed are not only specific to each type of cancer, but also to each person and their genetic makeup.

That's very important for us to understand when it comes to fitness as well. Current studies will almost always report an "average" result. They won't report the fact that a specific protocol helped 6 people, did nothing for 2, and hurt 2. They'll just say that it helped 6 out of 10. Unfortunately, all you can really do with results such as those is use them to design a future study, as the results generated more questions than answers.

To make matters worse, once the results get filtered through a few people with agendas (maybe reporters, but more often the people who funded the study), the only results that will get back to you are "it worked."

The last reason to not trust a lot of the info you read and are told is sad but true: Ego. It's pretty common practice even among experts and scientists to refuse to change their opinions on a subject even long after new evidence has proven the old theories incorrect.

I have read that quantum physics did not start to gain acceptance until after Einstein (with his relativistic theories) passed away. Yes, even the best and the brightest fall victim to ego. Many experts simply find it nearly impossible to admit something they've promoted and written about for years is simply incorrect or incomplete.

I see these errors all the time. When I'm reading the research journals and see useful or interesting conclusions, I make sure to always look at the data before I start using those conclusions.

If you've gotten offended by anything you've read so far, you might want to stop reading right now. Although all of the information in this book is backed not only by my personal experience, but also by the scientific research done by others, unfortunately, I've found many people are just not willing to listen to advice that runs counter to what they've been told by the "experts" in their lives.

I've actually had people get angry at me for giving them information or advice that they requested. Turns out, they didn't really want information, they just wanted confirmation that they were doing all they could do to meet their goals. Hence, their failure wasn't their own fault, it was genetics, or a busy schedule, or some other excuse. The last thing they wanted to hear was that if they wanted to accomplish their goals they needed to start from scratch.

I don't want to get into specific exercise recommendations in the opening pages, but I'll give you an example: Perhaps the biggest fitness error I see over and over and over again is the long-standing belief that if you want to be "fit" or thin, or healthy, you need to do cardio, cardio, and more cardio. Twenty years ago, it was so accepted that cardio is all you needed, that anyone who said otherwise was simply laughed off the stage.

This is such a prevalent belief that even today after many studies have shown that cardio is only a part of the fitness puzzle, many individuals still refuse to believe it. Part of it is just the fact that people don't like to change. Someone who has always based their entire fitness regimen on endless hours of mind numbing steady state cardio just doesn't want to hear that the reason they haven't aged as gracefully as they would have liked, or that they have bad knees from repetitive stress, is due to what they've been doing to themselves for the past fifteen years. But part of it is due to the fact that many people really don't like strenuous exercise, or exercise which requires any amount of concentration.

Over the years I cannot count the number of individuals who have simply refused to believe that 4 hours a week of a balanced program consisting of cardio, resistance training and flexibility along with a healthy diet will give them far superior results than 10 hours a week grinding out miles on the treadmill or elliptical.

Why Trust This Book?

So, why would you trust me? Very good question. Perhaps you shouldn't. Or at least don't take everything I say as gospel. I'm sure 10 years from now, most of my methods will be proven correct, but probably a few will not. I've certainly modified many of my ideas as new evidence becomes available. But unlike most of the "experts" out there, when I find new information, I have no problem admitting there is a better way.

An expert who is not open-minded and willing to alter their theories is really only an expert for a very short period of time.

Not only have I been a fitness expert, but I've also been a laboratory engineer and scientist. If you want someone to stand up on TV in brightly stripped tights and endorse some cheap fitness device that couldn't possibly do what it is advertised to do, then you have the wrong fitness guru. However, if you want one that has spent the last fifteen years reading and applying the latest health and fitness studies, then you're in the right place. You won't find a lot of people like me in the fitness industry, at least not outside of professional sports. In pro sports the cost of failure is so high that you will find people who really put in the time to know what they are doing.

So why not just go to a pro sports strength and conditioning specialist? Well, there are two problems with that. First you probably couldn't afford him even if he would "lower" himself to working with a mere mortal, but also, his knowledge is very specific to a very specialized class of individual. Professional athletes really are unique. The training they are capable of and willing to endure goes so far beyond what the average person can do that much of the training this type of coach would put you through would result in injury. Playing sports is an athlete's life and that difference alone makes any program designed for athletes almost irrelevant for you. You are probably looking for far less exacting results and are therefore less interested in spending every waking moment working on those goals.

Unlike these very competent pro sports trainers, I've worked with hundreds of individuals just like you. Busy professionals who value both their fitness and their time have always been my bread and butter. Also, since I started out as an out of shape teenager for whom none of the conventional wisdom ever worked, I've been in the same trenches many of you are in. I had to search out the necessary knowledge to turn bad genetics and bad (FDA endorsed) eating habits into new habits that would allow me to carve out the physique I now have. Like you, I had to fit my workouts in with a more than full-time job, and had to come up with a way of eating that fit within the confines of brown bag lunches, donuts in the break room, co-workers going for fast food every day, and business trips where I never knew where or when my next meal would be. I know the time constraints you have, and I know what you are probably willing to do, and what will probably make you want to quit the program altogether. I've been able to weed out the methods that just aren't worth the effort and maximize the effects of the time you do spend in the gym.

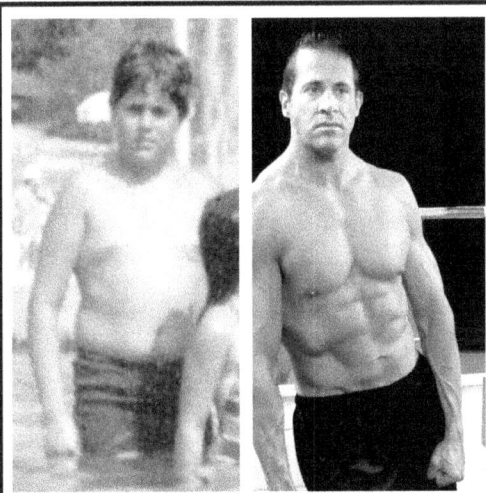

A lot of fitness "experts" either don't walk the walk, or they were genetically blessed and really don't know how they look the way they do. I didn't have the fortune of ever being naturally fit, and I've struggled (and succeeded) with it my entire life.

When I look at the programs some of my clients were on before coming to me, it's obvious why they failed to meet their goals. The unfortunate thing about the mainstream health and fitness industry is that the success of most programs is not judged by whether the user has long term success with their goals, but instead is either short term goal based or, even worse, based not on results at all but on how fun or easy the program is. In some cases, these programs do generate results, but at the cost of sacrificing much of the client's life. One recently popular program, although very colorful and not bad as far as results are concerned, is so time-consuming that I can't imagine anyone in the real world following it for longer than a couple of months.

I have, on occasion, run into ex-clients several months after they left my program. They'll say something like "I decided to switch to XXX program (insert a fancy European sounding term for xxx). I know your program works for a lot of people, but I like this program. It works for me." I'm pretty observant, and I can quickly deduce by the ten pounds they've put back on, and the bad postural habits that have already started to come back, what they really mean is "This program is easy and entertaining and that is what I was really looking for. Now I can tell my friends I'm paying a lot for an expensive exercise program, so it can't be my fault I still look and feel terrible."

On the other end of the spectrum, some people seem to want to take the "if a little isn't working, just do more" approach to exercise or diet. If spending an hour, four times a week on the treadmill isn't getting them where they want to be, then do two hours, six times a week. If a 1200 calories per day low fat diet isn't working, cut it to 1000.

The problem is, this rarely works, and it's terribly inefficient. Doing more of something that isn't working is never a good solution to any problem. You need to reevaluate your methods, and maybe even start from scratch.

The efficiency or small amount of time necessary, is where I feel my methods really shine. I, and many of my long term clients, often get the "if I could only spend my entire life working out like you do" line from people around them. It's always a nice comfortable excuse to think that you simply don't have time to be in shape. They always look at us in stunned disbelief when we tell them we workout only 4 or 5 hours a week. Compare that to the 20 hours the average American spends watching TV each week and you start to realize that it truly is a poor excuse.

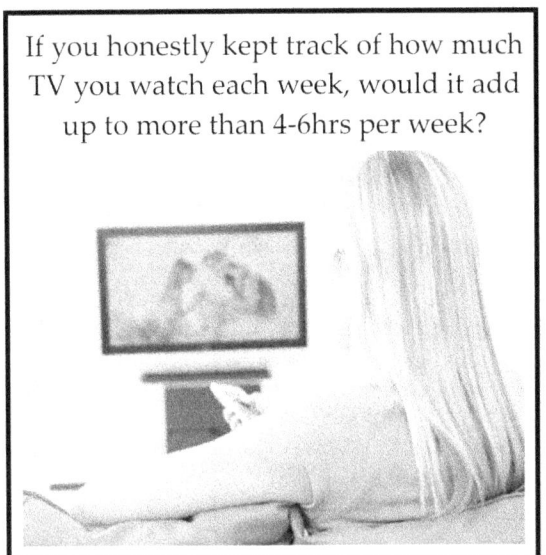

If you honestly kept track of how much TV you watch each week, would it add up to more than 4-6hrs per week?

Chapter 2 – Fitness Philosophy

Fitness is 95% mental. Yes, I know you've heard that before about a lot of things in life, and it's because, more often than not, it's true.

It's unfortunate that sometimes it seems to take a therapist, more than a trainer to help someone on their road to fitness. Before I would take on a new client, I would start with a one to two hour consultation. After doing it for so long, I can sometimes tell someone within minutes whether they will succeed or fail in their fitness goals. Sometimes the consultation would end up as a two hour back and forth with them assuring me they really could do it.

When people find out what I do, they always want to tell me about their latest workout program, and often, why it's better than anything I offer. Of course they never really want advice, and I almost always bite my tongue, but it usually doesn't take more than a few sentences for me to make a pretty accurate prediction of their possibility for success.

It's not just the systems and methods that they have chosen, that tell me what I need to know, but also how they talk about their new fitness goals, and the expectations they have. What were their excuses in the past, and what's really changed? Are they really resolved to not letting "life" give them the same excuses three months from now?

Are their aspirations permanent, or just fleeting whims that will disappear as quickly as they arrived? We'll talk more about excuses later, but if this individual is talking about their new fitness program in any way that leads me to believe that the change is only temporary, then they're obviously just setting themselves up for failure. A fitness program is never easier than it is in the beginning when you're excited about the process. Once that excitement has worn off, if you're not mentally "there" then the excuses will start flowing.

There are sometimes temporary reasons to get in shape. The bride that wants to fit into the special wedding dress, or the ex high school football player who wants to look like "he's still got it" for his buddies at the reunion, but those really aren't the people for whom I'm writing this book. I'm writing this for those of you that realize your health and fitness is so important that it needs to be a permanent part of your life.

Just like you'd never say "I'm way too busy to brush my teeth for the next couple of months," you need to get to the point where finding excuses to stop working out seem just as ridiculous. Whether it's your teeth, or your muscles, bones, heart, etc, maintaining the body you were given is just too important.

Your goals are also critical. Are they realistic, or more importantly, is the time you've set aside and the plan you've setup to achieve these goals realistic? Nothing will deflate your mental drive as much as getting a couple months into a program, only to realize you've really just been spinning your wheels.

The Definition of Fitness

Most controversies would soon be ended, if those engaged in them would first accurately define their terms, and then adhere to their definitions. - Tryon Edwards

It is not the end of the physical body that should worry us. Rather, our concern must be to live while we're alive. - Elisabeth Kubler-Ross

Avoiding death or enjoying life?

When you are reading my ideas on health and fitness, you have to realize my core belief system is a little different from mainstream society's. The world we live in, anchored mainly by conventional medicine, defines health as the lack of death. It doesn't take much observation to figure that out. Our health insurance will pay almost any amount of money to keep you from dying, but next to nothing to keep you healthy. If you are elderly, on the verge of death and in pain, our system will make sure to keep you in pain and on this earth as long as is humanly possible.

I think you can see where I'm going with this. My opinion is that health and fitness have more to do with quality of life than the length of time we stay alive. Not that I don't want to live a long life as well, but I understand how uncertain that can be, and I'd rather spend 60 vibrant years on this earth than 30 vibrant years followed by 50 years declining into incapacity. I truly hope someone has the compassion to NOT let me sit on life support and medication for months or years after my fate has been laid before me.

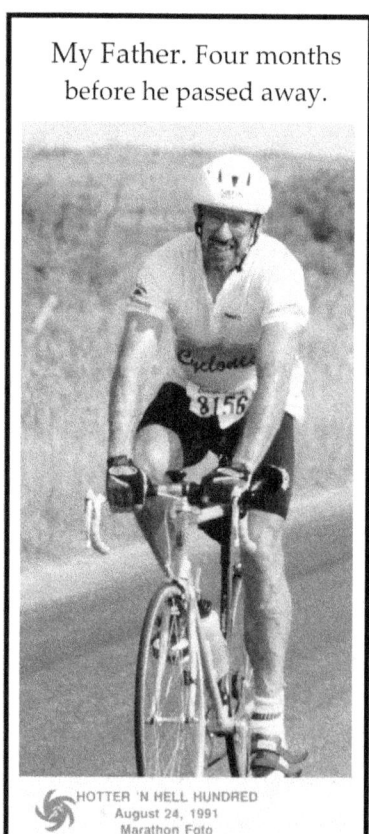

My Father. Four months before he passed away.

HOTTER 'N HELL HUNDRED
August 24, 1991
Marathon Foto

We all have events in our lives that shape our thoughts and opinions, and I'm no different. My grandfather was typical of many at the time - a moderate drinker, smoker and modestly overweight. He died at 57 of a heart attack. My father spent most of his life trying to avoid his father's fate. He ate the government recommended healthy diet, worked out, ran marathons, didn't smoke or drink, maintained a healthy weight....and died at 56 of a heart attack.

You may say I'm unduly prejudiced by this unfortunate part of my past (my father was, and always will be the single most positive influence on the man I am today), but the fact remains, whether it's a heart attack or being hit by a car, our existence on this earth is tenuous. Not that I'm going to ignore the value of behaviors that will help me live a longer life, it's just that when given the choice between a workout or diet habit that may or may not extend my life and one that will definitely improve the quality of my life, I will almost always choose the later.

This is a fact you must be aware of when reading this material. It makes some, but not all of my advice very specific to those who feel as I do. I will always try to be specific as to which goal each recommendation is intended for. Most, but not all of my recommendations will really apply to overall health and fitness, whether judged by length or quality of life, but there are many more theories on longevity that may be much more specific to living to the oldest possible age with no regard to quality of life.

Many dietary theorists claim that near starvation diets on a continual basis are path to a long life. Of course, this requires looking like a stick figure, nearly concentration camp thin. You can forget about vigorous activities like mountain biking or skiing, and you may have to worry about bone strength later in life. I personally don't feel the many quality of life sacrifices are worth it. You may disagree. I've also read a theory lately (published as a front page article in Time Magazine) that if you want to live a long life, you should avoid any sort of strenuous exercise at all....walking, maybe a little easy stretching, but definitely no intense weight workouts, sprints or intervals.

I won't argue that the many broken bones and torn ligaments I've suffered from my habit of playing dangerous sports more aggressively than my capabilities allow, are not the best way to ensure longevity. However, I also feel nonaggressive methods to a long life will not allow the body to maintain the strong muscles and bones that are so necessary for quality of life as we age.

I'm not talking about the conventional definition of quality of life, where all fun active sporting activities are done and over well before 50. A walking cane is not uncommon by 60, a wheel chair by 70 and dementia long before 80. What I'm talking about is Jack Lelanne type quality of life. I'm talking about a level of health and fitness that doesn't have to decline drastically as we age.

When I was in my early twenties, the 30 year olds in my office said things like "just wait till you hit your 30's". When I hit thirty, the '40 Something's' said "just wait till you hit 40" Now that I'm in my forties, and look 30, I've got 38 year olds saying "just wait till you're my age!" Yes, on at least a dozen occasions I've had people much younger than I say that in all seriousness. If I make it that long, I can't wait till I'm 80, and the 70 year olds are saying "wait till you get to my age."

Many women will say "Yeah, a guy can do that, but it's different for women." While I can't argue that society views wrinkles differently on women than men, our bodies are much more similar. Women can maintain a smoking hot physique late into life, just as easily as a guy can. She just needs to follow similar methods, something very few do.

Muscle – Fountain of Youth?

If you haven't figured it out by now, I feel adding and maintaining muscle is critical to almost all long term health and fitness goals. First, muscle allows us to do whatever it is we want to do. The more healthy muscle we have (to a point) the more we can do. Although most of you have no desire to have enough muscle to pull a locomotive with a rope like a "strongman" competitor, the lack of muscle in most older individuals is by far the biggest factor in the decline of the quality of life. From the ability to dance at your grandkids wedding, climb stairs, get up out of a chair or even move around without the assistance of a wheel chair, muscle is most often the key.

The human body adds muscle tissue as the body grows through the teenage years. Depending on activity level, all of us will have a good deal of muscle in our early twenties. For many people, weight maintenance at that age, is only a matter of cutting out some junk food and doing some cardio. Many of you already know how that doesn't seem to work once you reach your late thirties or early forties.

You see, the body knows that muscle tissue is highly inefficient, and it is. It takes a lot of calories to maintain muscle tissue and thousands of years ago, evolution did not reward an individual who carried around more muscle than necessary, so starting in our mid twenties, our bodies start to get rid of any muscle that we aren't using.

Evolutionarily, it was also not a good thing to have a bunch of virile 80 year olds running around. Yes, one way or another, your body is trying to kill you. Declining hormone levels and decreasing muscle tissue is nature's way of making sure our species doesn't have a bunch of older people running around making babies they won't live to take care of.

However this isn't "thousands of years ago." The ability to burn extra calories is no longer a bad thing as food and calories are now plentiful. More on the calorie burning abilities of muscle later, but for now, let's just say that keeping the muscle you had when you were young or even adding a little is absolutely best way to maintain your body fat level and quality of life as you age.

Some of you may have managed to maintain your weight as you age, just by adjusting how much you eat. However, if you do manage to maintain your body weight as you age, without any resistance training, you are still losing muscle, and replacing it with fat. Eventually the declining ability to burn calories will catch up to you, as will the fact that at the same weight, since you have less muscle and more fat. You will look less "toned" and fit.

This is true for both men and women. There is such a stigma against muscle growth in women, that many times it's very difficult to convince women that this is so essential for them. You are not going to "turn into a man" or grow big muscles "like a female bodybuilder". Both male and female bodybuilders have one thing in common that you don't: Testosterone. Men have it naturally and male AND female bodybuilders can get it through a needle, but both have far more of it than you ever will. You are not going to get huge, and even if by some genetic mutation you started to get more muscular than you want, all it will take is backing off on the workouts and you'll lose that extra muscle in no time.

Bulk is Not Muscle

Let's make sure we understand that I'm talking about muscle, not "bulk". Getting bulky is usually the result of diet and body fat gain, not muscle gain. I have, over the years, worked with perhaps a half dozen women who were really genetically blessed, such that they had an easy time putting on muscle without drugs. However, even in these half dozen cases, the only time they looked bulky or overly muscular, was when they didn't have their diet under control. When their diet, and hence their body fat levels were where they wanted them to be, they were fit, trim, and what most would refer to as "toned".

Let's define a term that many people misuse. "Toned" is simply a state of low body fat and sufficient muscle. You will frequently hear people say things like "I don't want to put on muscle, I just want to be toned." Unfortunately there is no such thing as small toned muscles, your muscles will be whatever size they are, and the ability to see them will be controlled by the level of body fat you have. If you have an example of someone who you feel is very "toned" chances are they have moderately more muscle than the average person (not too much more), and lower body fat than your average person.

There are other factors that affect what terms people will use to describe you at a given fitness level, however other than the amount of muscle and amount of body fat, most of the other factors are genetic, and without surgery, are next to impossible to alter. How tall you are, how long each section of your legs and arms are, and the attachment and insertion points for each muscle will give each individual a different look with the same amount of muscle, but you're not going to change these factors. Yes, the commercials are blatantly lying to you when they say their brand of Pilates will give you long, lean muscles, like a dancer. Dancers have long lean muscles because they are dancers, or perhaps they are dancers because they have long, lean muscles, who knows which came first, the chicken or the egg, but certainly not the pilates.

But back to muscle. It is the SINGLE MOST IMPORTANT FACTOR influencing your metabolism, appearance as you age, and quality of life. It is unfortunate that society has convinced many men and the vast majority of women that their bodies have to grow soft and weak as they age. Lose skin that hangs off your arms, the cellulite on your thighs, and the general feeling that your body is just not as "tight" as it used to be, even though you may weigh the same, it is ALL due to decreasing muscle mass, and it CAN be prevented or reversed.

A pound of fat is a LOT bigger (and lumpier) than a pound of muscle. Yes, it is possible to put on muscle and look smaller at the same time!

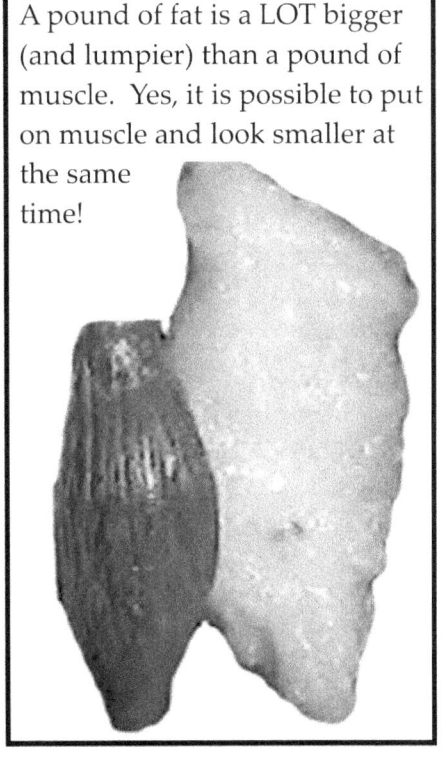

Remember, I'm not talking about the feel or appearance of your skin. For some of you it may be hard for you to accept that something like cellulite is more a factor of what goes on below the skin, but it is. Certainly, someone blessed with very elastic skin will have less of an appearance of cellulite but the fundamental cause of most of what we don't like about our bodies as we age is body fat and muscle related, not due to the skin that covers it. Certainly there are theories for keeping the skin young and healthy, but you'll need to look elsewhere for that information.

I'm also not talking about female breasts either. There is no chest workout that will firm up your breasts after a couple of children. Unlike the rest of your body, breasts are entirely body fat supported by skin. Life does take its toll there.

I am noticing a trend in even younger women now days. Whereas in the past, simply being 20 and not being overweight assured you of a reasonably toned physique. However, recently, ridiculous cyclic dieting at a very young age, along with extended cardio and a complete lack of any resistance exercise are resulting in the same thin but flabby appearance (we call it the "thin fat" look) you might have previously expected only in the 40+ generation.

We'll leave this topic behind with one last observation. IT IS NEVER TOO LATE!! A 45-year-old can put on a little muscle and that flabby appearance (and cellulite) will be greatly reduced or even disappear completely. A 85 year old can see their quality of life improve tremendously in as little as a couple of months!

Goals

"Failing to plan is planning to fail." - Alan Lakein

The first thing I always do when meeting with a new client is ask "What are your goals?" They'll say "I want to be in shape" or "I want to be fit". I know I'm going to hear something meaningless and general like that, and I'm prepared with a whole new set of questions. I might ask "What do you mean by 'in shape'?"

Or they might be a little more honest and say "I want to look hot in a bikini again." In which case I'll ask "Why?"

For me, as their new trainer, it was important to really establish their true goals. In most cases, I'd have to ask three or four sets of progressively deeper questions to get at what really brought them to me. That was very important for me as sometimes, the reason they first stated really had nothing to do with the real reason.

For instance, he may have told me "I want to be fit." But after digging for a while it came out that his wife had recently lost 20 pounds and was getting a lot of looks from other guys. She works in an office with a lot of younger guys and my new client was very worried he was going to lose her if he didn't shape up.

As a trainer, my job is 50% therapist, so the value of knowing what the real motivation is can't be underestimated. The same is true if you are your own trainer. At one point or another, we've all "lied to ourselves." Starting an exercise program may sound like a minor thing, but the fact is, if it's to be successful, it will be life changing and lifelong.

If you don't start out being honest with yourself about your goals, you will not be nearly as happy with the results as you'd be with very clear goals and a plan of action that is tailored to those goals.

Even if you really do want to "get in shape" or "get fit," what does "in shape" or "fit" really mean. I've found it means COMPLETLY different things to different people. As I write this section, I'm spending the weekend at an Ironman. I've noticed this is a major step up from the last marathon I attended. Many of the participants at least have some sort of lean muscle mass, unlike long distance runners, who look weak and sickly and will likely suffer for their hobby in old age.

Yet, on the other end of the spectrum, I've known many competitive power lifters who, although they were incredibly strong, many of them couldn't walk up a flight of stairs without pausing to catch their breath. Or, how about Bodybuilders who have bodies that ripple with muscle like some Greek god, yet, would have a hard time keeping up in just about any sport that required movement, and whose blood test results would scare even the most jaded physician.

I'm not trying to put down any of these individuals. Quite the contrary, I have great respect for each of them. However, each of them eats and works out for very specific goals. The same is true for you, the average non-competitive, non-athlete. When you say: "I want to be fit" you're probably setting yourself up for failure. You need to realize that certain exercise programs that most would say are classic ways to "get fit" are really only going to accomplish a very limited subset of your real goals.

What I'm saying is that if your REAL goal is to look better, then just admit it and define exactly how you'd like to look. You'll waste a lot less time than if you follow a program more appropriate to someone training for a half marathon. And if you're goal is to be healthy as you age, you might want a program that is concerned with the health of your entire body and not just your heart.

"I Just Want To Workout"

You might say, "I just want to work out, I don't want to have to think about goals." This would seem like a no-brainer, but you don't know how many times I've heard clients say "I've achieved the goals I came here to achieve, so now I just want to work out and not worry about goals." This usually means they also don't want to bother with the bi-monthly fitness evaluation either. In almost every case, within six months they've regressed significantly.

You're either moving forwards or moving backwards. If you don't have a fitness goal, no matter how minor, and you're not continuing to monitor your fitness level, I can almost assure you that your overall fitness level will decrease.

I've even seen it in myself: I know I don't have the talent to be a professional athlete, I feel terrible if I'm much below 8 percent body fat, and every time I try to up my bench-press, deadlift or squat much beyond my current level, I end up hurting myself (from overreaching and dumb errors on my part, not the exercises themselves). So every once in a while I catch myself without any real goals. I'm happy with my fitness level, I'm getting positive comments from others, I'm strong, healthy, and fit even if I'll never be a pro athlete, or model on the cover of "Men's Fitness."

Then it happens: I catch myself just going through the motions. My workouts get lazy, and my diet deteriorates. Pretty soon I'm looking at myself in the mirror and not liking what I see. That's when I have to reset my goals and get back on track.

Realistic Goals and Methods

It should go without saying that goals have to be realistic. Deciding that your goal is to lose 50 pounds before your trip to Cancun in two months is just setting yourself up for failure. Some people say you need to reach for the moon in order to accomplish anything, but I feel that reaching for the moon only works if you're NASA. If you're anyone else, reaching for the moon results in a fiery crash and burn! You need to set realistic goals.

While writing this I ran into a friend at a party. I asked her where her boyfriend was, and she said he stayed at home because he was four weeks into a very popular exercise program, couldn't drink alcohol, and hence didn't want to be tempted. You may be saying "Good for him!" and I do truly wish him the best, but with that one statement alone I was pretty certain he was doomed to long term failure. Or, I should say, the program doomed him.

It's not that giving up alcohol is a bad thing, it's just that he was obviously doing something temporary. Something that he was not going to stick with long term, because it's not that drinking alcohol was ever a problem for him, and he was certainly not going to give up being social forever. Because the program itself is not, by its very nature, a program that was designed for long term adherence, he is doomed for failure.

I know that he is an intelligent, hard working individual, but by using this overly ambitious program, I can predict with a high degree of confidence, that within a couple months he will be right back to where he started.

I know this is a hard point for many of you to understand. You're probably saying "What's wrong with making a temporary sacrifice in order to meet a goal?" Nothing at all as long as the goal is only temporary as well! It's one thing to cut back on the calories a little, or up the workout intensity a bit in order to lose the initial weight, but if your goals are long term (as they should be, who wants to be fit for a month or two?), you're methods need to be long term as well.

Conflicting Goals

You also need to make sure you don't set conflicting goals: A beginner may put on some muscle while they are losing fat but you'll have much better luck if you just try for one goal at a time. Also, watch the timing of your goals. Setting a realistic weight loss goal around a trip to the beach is a great idea, but trying to continue to lose weight while on that Caribbean cruise may be a bit unrealistic. A more realistic goal may be to limit your total weight gain to only a pound, since you know you're not going to be able to resist the buffets and margaritas.

It also helps a lot to have long, medium and short term goals. What the sports performance world calls macro, messo and microcycles. For an athlete, a long term goal or macrocycle might be winning a Gold at the Olympics in two years. For you it might be getting into the same shape as you were when you were 20 by this time next year. An athlete might have a medium term goal of improving his anaerobic capacity, and you might have the same goal but with the intent of upping the amount of work you can do in every workout, thereby increasing long term fat loss. A short term or micro cycle for an athlete might be a two week workout plan that would change every two weeks and your short term goal might also be completing the two week workout/nutrition plan that will be necessary to move you towards the weight loss.

Short Term Goals

For many of us, having short term workout plans is a little tough. Many fitness experts will go so far as to say that you need to know exactly what you're going to do in the gym every workout, and those workouts should be planned well ahead of time. That may work for some professional athletes (although I question this), but for those of us in the real world it does help to at least plan your workouts, even if you deviate from the plan as often as not.

"Life" does get in the way. You may plan to get to the gym Monday, Wednesday, Friday, and Saturday, but if a major client at work needs 20 hours from you on Wednesday, you may need to move that workout to Thursday. That change in timing may also alter Friday's workout. In fact, the long hours may also result in less intensity both days, with the result that you will have to make up for it with extra intensity the next time you are fully recovered.

This type of short term planning does require that you know your own body, and that you are honest with yourself. There will be days when you will have more energy and be able to put in a more intense workout. You're much better off taking advantage of that than trying to stick to some arbitrary workout schedule.

It really does help to know "What am I doing this week?", "What easily foreseeable goal do I have for the next month or two?", and finally, "Where do I see myself in two years?"

What if you really are satisfied with your fitness level? To be honest, I find that hard to believe. Almost all of us have something we'd like to improve. Or maybe it's something you always wanted to be able to do, but never could. Like dunking a basketball or doing 10 chin-ups. Maybe you're pretty happy with the way you look but you've always wanted more defined abs, or better calves. These may seem like minor or silly goals, but as long as you actually HAVE a goal at all, you will be more motivated and your workout more intense.

A couple of summers ago, I noticed that photos of myself in a swimsuit looked slightly less fit than the year before. Many people would say "I'm in my 40's, I can't expect to look this way forever", but instead, I set a goal of doing a photo shoot the next summer, where I was determined to look better than ever. It may sound narcissistic, but the fact is, the thought of the upcoming photo shoot energized my workouts for months. I not only looked better than ever, but also felt more physically fit in general than I had in years. I now do this at the beginning of every summer.

Overachieving Your Goals

Warning! Blatant personal rant ahead! Yes, it is opinion only, but one backed by many years of observations, and conversations with men and women of all levels of fitness.

I'm not a big fan of many of the psychological terms used to describe otherwise normal behavior, but "Body Dismorphia" is very real, if overused. Body Dismorphia is a disorder in which the affected person is excessively concerned about and preoccupied by a perceived defect in his or her physical features. Just as there are many obese individuals who simply do not view themselves as being as overweight as they are, and anorexics that will always view themselves as overweight even when you can see their ribs, many fitness enthusiasts take their personal fitness beyond what they had initially intended.

Certainly, if you have the genetics to be a professional bodybuilder or fitness competitor, and you want to set that as your goal, then you will have to gain muscle and drop body fat to a level far beyond anything required for fitness, health, or physical appearance. However, if those are not your goals, make sure you're always keeping your real goals in mind.

I know countless individuals, who got so caught up in the pursuit of fitness that they went far beyond their goals. Both men and women, who had the desire to be perceived as fit and attractive, got their first "Wow, I love your arms" compliment and went off the deep end. Although they will still swear they only want to be fit and attractive, they take themselves to a level of musculature and/or lack of body fat that is no longer considered attractive to the vast majority of society. Examples are guys who can't scratch their own back or fitness enthusiasts who pursue low body fat to the point of visible ribs and boney shoulders. It always helps to have someone else that you trust to evaluate how you are progressing. I have several friends and other professional in the

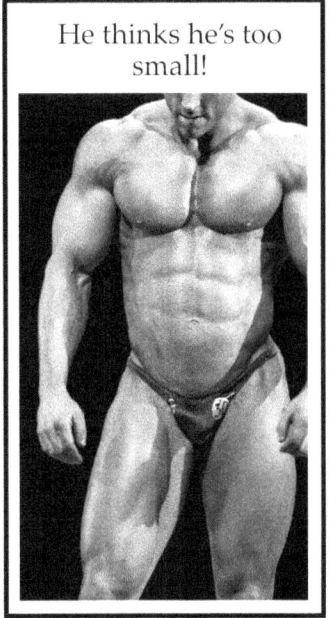

He thinks he's too small!

industry that I have evaluate my physique for symmetry, posture, and overall balance.

I'm not trying to tell you what your goals should be. If you started off just wanting to be fit enough to be healthy and look good in a bathing suit, but in the process, got so addicted to the pursuit of strength that your goals changed, then fine, go for it, but make sure your real goals are what you say they are. End of rant.

There's a reason one of the first questions I ask someone when I talk to them about fitness is "What are your goals?" It may be cliché, but if you're failing to plan you're planning to fail.

Consistency

If there is one rule to health and fitness that completely dominates all others, and by such a wide margin that nothing else comes close, it's consistency.

Not that you can do everything wrong and still make progress if you just spend time in the gym, but you can make a lot of mistakes and still have the body you want as long as you're willing to put in the effort day in and day out, year after year.

It Takes Time – But it's Worth it!

Being very fit does not require that you live in the gym, or that you abandon all food with taste. However, it does require consistency of both diet and workouts. Most people don't want to hear it when I tell them just how long it will be before they reach their fitness goals, but the reality is that there are no quick fixes. Yes, there is surgery, but if you really want to look and feel great, it may take some time. One of the biggest lies told in the fitness and weight loss industries is the time required to achieve your goals. Let's be honest, unless it only took you 12 weeks to get out of shape, it's not going to take you 12 weeks to get back into shape. I have yet to see one single case of anyone making a large transformation in a short time, other than someone who was very recently in great shape and just let themselves go.

In fact, most of the Before/After transformation photos you see are very specifically fitness models who did just that. For the very purpose of making money from Before/After transformations they allowed themselves to put on weight that they knew they could quickly drop. There are even people who specialize in Before/After photography and can even do photo shoots of the same person on the very same day, and make it look like a dramatic transformation.

One very big supplement company is well known for a series of ads they ran with a pregnant fitness model. The shots were taken to make it look like she was just out of shape and then they claimed her sudden weight loss was due to their diet supplement and not simply the birth of her baby.

And that's another thing that separates me from the rest of the health and fitness industry. I'm not going to lie to you. As difficult as the road has been, I've never tried to succeed in the fitness industry with anything other than genuinely effective fitness programs. It may be much easier to make money with fads and gimmicks, but that just isn't me. It wasn't when I was a trainer, and it certainly isn't now that I am an author and consultant.

In fact, for once, this works to my advantage. There are so many other health and fitness books that ARE NOT willing to tell you the truth that hopefully mine stands out to those of you ready to "handle the truth."

Many of my thoughts on health and fitness may be depressing to many people, but most will spend longer delaying the decision to get in shape than they would just making it happen. If your goals are going to take five years to accomplish, that doesn't mean you're not going to look and feel much better after four months, it just means your ultimate goals are going to take some time. But I guarantee, when you look back on it five years from now, you will not regret the decision. What seemed like a lot of work back when you started will end up being a change in lifestyle that will not only make the end worthwhile, but the journey will be a reward in itself.

How Long?

So how long will it take you to accomplish your goals? There are a ton of factors that go into that, and if I could sit down with each one of you, I could give you a really good idea, but it's not as if I can really give you a mathematical formula. One good way to estimate is to ask yourself how long it took you to get out of shape. When someone is simply trying to get back to where they were at a younger age, then it probably will take about the same length of time it took you to get out of shape. This does not count the time you may have spent yo-yoing back and forth, or the periods of time when you may have maintained your condition, but just how many months of combined neglect it took to get to where you are now.

But we can get a little more specific. Weight loss is certainly the number one fitness goal. Although there are all sorts of stories of people losing 100 pounds in six months, that's the exception, not the rule. Not only is it very difficult, but depending on the weight you are starting at, could be dangerous, and probably not productive to your long term goals.

Some general rules of thumb are as follows: If you do everything right, and you are starting more than 100 lbs over your target weight, you could expect to lose 2-3 lbs per week to start. Once you get down to within 50-80 lbs of your target weight, 2 lbs per week is more reasonable. At 20lbs from your target weight, you may find it tough to lose more than a pound a week.

Of course this all depends on where you started, and how long you were overweight. Someone who has just let themselves go for a few years (less than five) is probably going to find that the weight comes off more easily than it will for someone who has been at that weight for 10 or more years. Your body will not have adapted to a new "norm" as it will if you've been overweight for longer.

Never neglect the "mental" aspects. Although it really does come down to the science of eating and exercise, it's not always easy to follow the plan. In fact sometimes it's nearly an insurmountable challenge. You WILL make mistakes. You have to plan for them to some degree. The longer you have been overweight, the more your body will fight the weight loss, and the more mistakes you will probably make. You'll have good weeks and bad weeks, so even if you are shooting for three pounds a week, you should be incredibly happy to average two pounds per week.

It will be even tougher if you were overweight and inactive as a child and teen. There's obviously nothing you can do about this (other than make sure your children don't suffer the same fate), but if you were overweight as you grew up, your body will have manufactured more fat cells than someone who grew up at a normal weight. Your body will always be trying to keep these cells full, and it will always be tougher to lose weight. To compound the problem, if you were also inactive, you will find you will burn a lot fewer calories in your workouts. After working with hundreds of clients, I've seen a very strong trend: People who were active and athletic in their youth are simply able to work out harder sooner in the program. More on diet and exercise for youth later.

The point is, there are no quick fixes. If you plan to start "getting in shape" plan to make it a lifelong goal. Even if you reach your goals, you can never stop. Why would you get in shape, just to let yourself go? You have to look at this as a lifestyle change. As I stated earlier, would you ever stop brushing your teeth? Well, that's how you have to look at working out. It's body maintenance, and something we all need to do, regardless of our age. You can think of it as a journey, not a destination, if you'd like. I don't know anyone who has ever regretted the journey.

Excuses

Please don't let the following topic get you down. Yes, I'm going to beat up on you a little. Some of you may want to put the book down, but do yourself a favor and try to read it with an open mind. This is a VERY important topic.

A couple of the various dictionary definitions of "excuse" are: Act of seeking to remove the blame of, serve as an apology or justification for, release from an obligation or duty, seek or obtain exemption or release for (oneself).

"Justification" "seek release" "remove the blame of" "an apology of justification for". Notice any common trend? An excuse is just that, an excuse.

I've been in the position to hear just about every excuse imaginable for why someone can't get in shape. I can only recall once instance of someone having an excuse that was actually relevant for their lack of progress, and that was a horrendous auto accident that left the client with back problems that no one (including me) could seem to help her with. Other than that, every excuse I've heard (including all the other "my back hurts" excuses) was just a reason to fail.

I've heard it all: "I don't have time." "My kids come first." "I don't have money to join a gym." "I've got an injury or illness." "My doctor says I shouldn't work out because (fill in the blank with any of a number of supposed illnesses)." "I'm traveling too much right now." "My husband likes me just the way I am." "I never know when I'm going to be called into work, and can't ever get a workout schedule setup." Etc. etc. etc.

But for every excuse, I've met someone who had the given situation much worse than the excuse holder, yet somehow managed to overcome and accomplish their goals.

I have a good friend who is just a great person in so many ways. He's smart, educated, hard working, caring, etc., but about once a month, he says something like "Starting next month I'm going to start working out for sure. I just need to wait until ____ (fill in the blank with this month's excuse)." I politely humor him (most of the time), but the fact is, getting in shape is just not a priority to him. Since he has a gym at home, as well as at work, pretty much every excuse he comes up with sounds really lame. I'm sure if he ever listened to a tape recording of himself, he'd be a little embarrassed. It's not as if I ever pressure him to workout. Whatever shape he's in doesn't affect our friendship in the least, but somehow he seems to need the excuses instead of just being honest with himself and saying "I'm fine with how I look and feel, and being in better shape is just not a priority".

I actually have a certain amount of respect for a person who is out of shape but honest with themselves. If an overweight person says to me "Yeah, I know I'm a heart attack waiting to happen but I like who I am, and I enjoy food and my free time too much to diet and exercise." I'm not saying I endorse that attitude, but at least this guy knows where he stands. He's not making excuses, he's just not interested in change.

When I would speak to a prospective client on the phone before they came in for a consultation, I would always ask: "Is there any reason you can't start the program right now?" This probably always sounded self-serving, as why would I waste time with someone who isn't ready to start, but it was a very important point: If they've got an excuse why they can't start now, they will just come up with another excuse later. When you have decided you are ready to get in shape, there are no relevant excuses. You start today. I've never seen it work any other way.

Sometimes, I would meet with a prospective client and quite bluntly tell them "You have too many excuses in your head already. You've already justified your failure." I would send them out the door as politely as possible, but I already knew (beyond any reasonable doubt) that they were going to fail. If they had learned anything from our talk, these same people would come back six months later and say "Ok, I'm done with the excuses. I realized just how right you were, and I decided my health is worth it. How soon can we start?" not "I took care of that situation and I'm ready to start now." If there's a reason (excuse) why you can't workout now, there will be another reason why you can't later either.

We talk about time, and how little it actually takes to get in shape later, but the other excuses are just as bad:

Family

"My kids come first." What kind of an example is it for your children if you can't make the time to stay in shape? Do you really want to die of a heart attack before you even get to enjoy seeing them grow up, get married, have children of their own, etc.? Get out there and be active WITH your kids. Modify the way the whole family eats, so that everyone is a healthy weight. Set up a cheap gym in the basement. Yes, I know, for each of these suggestions there's another excuse. I can't count the number of times I've heard parents say "In this day and age you can't NOT feed the family fast food." Using your kids as an excuse for being overweight or out of shape is probably one of the worst ones out there.

Money

"I don't have money to join a gym." There are a lot of REALLY good deals out there on gym memberships! I'm sure every one of you has at least one bad habit that costs more than a gym membership. Besides, your own body weight along with a few cheap dumbbells that you can easily store in a corner of the closet is all you REALLY need to get in shape.

Medical Condition

"I've got an injury or illness" or "My doctor says I shouldn't work out because...." These are particularly annoying. I can't count the number of times clients have actually brought a doctor's note in saying that because of some aliment, they can't workout. Let me let you in on a little secret: There are VERY few medical conditions where inactivity is recommended. If your doctor is willing to write you a note that says you should sit on your butt because your wrist hurts from typing too much at work, then, in my opinion, your doctor should have his/her license revoked. Exercise is almost always not only good for the entire body, but in many cases, is actually good for a particular injury (if done properly).

In every single case where I have received a doctor's note saying their patient should not work out, I have always gone online and/or talked with other experts. I have yet to find a single case where the doctor who wrote the letter had even a single shred of justification for the recommendation. In many cases, I found very specific evidence recommending that a patient with that condition continue being active.

You might say "What harm does it do to take a little time off while an injury or illness heals?" That may be true for a week or so if the injury or illness is acute. But that's not what these people were after. These were individuals who were making progress with their goals and for whatever reason, were looking for an excuse to quit. And the medical doctor gave it to them!!

Certainly if you have an acute illness that is requiring your immune system's uninterrupted attention to cure, of if there is broken bone that is so precarious that any activity at all could aggravate the injury, then sure, take a break. But that is rarely the case for more than a week. At various times in my life I have had injuries and illness including a broken leg, severely sprained and broken ankle, crushed collar bone, broken nose, broke almost every bone in one hand, broken rib, severely pulled groin, Pertussis, Mono, severe sinus infections, etc. etc. I can't recall one time where I stayed out of the gym more than a week. With the exception of the time I broke the collar bone in the midst of a getting a new home ready to move into, I've never regretted getting back into the gym (and in that occasion it wasn't the gym that hurt me, it was the hammering at home).

You can almost ALWAYS find a way to work around an injury.

Travel

"I'm traveling too much for work." This is certainly a hard one. You never know what kind of facilities you're going to find, you may be putting in very long hours while you're there, travel itself is tiring and will throw you off. No doubt about it, it's tough to stay in shape if you have to travel a lot, but I've seen too many people make it work.

When a client travels, they make sure to prioritize a

I've done my share of traveling and I know how tough it is to eat right and exercise while on the road.

workout at some point in the day regardless of what else is scheduled. Before and after the trip they get in extra tough workouts so that a little rest on the trip isn't a bad thing (this works especially well if you only travel for a few days a time), and they bring along protein powder and protein bars.

I don't want to make it sound like life is easy, and that any of these excuse doesn't make it tough to achieve your goals, but as with any other goal worth doing, if it's a high enough priority, you WILL find a way around them.

Hopefully you're still with me, and will give this topic some thought the next time even the toughest excuse comes up to allow you to stop working out. Again I'll say it: This has got to be like brushing your teeth. You wouldn't let something stop you from maintaining healthy teeth, why stop maintaining the rest of your body.

Walking into the Free Weights Section

This topic isn't just for women, but it's overwhelmingly an issue for so many women that I don't think labeling it that way is unfair. As you read on in this book, what will become obvious is that I strongly feel that the way the vast majority of women workout is virtually a waste of their time! This is not an understatement, and I feel it goes all the way to defining how society thinks of aging: Men can age gracefully and as long as they workout regularly, they can stay fit and attractive well into their later years, but women will get flabby and unattractive regardless of what they do. HORSEPUCKY!!

The problem is that women have this perception that exercise is all about how much cardio they can do, while most men will give some priority to some form of resistance training. I realize this bias exists because extra muscle is socially acceptable or even desirable for guys but not necessarily for women. However, as we've discussed and will continue to discuss, the only substantial difference between a 20-year-old and a 50-year-old man OR woman (from a function, appearance and metabolism standpoint) is the amount of muscle they carry. Ok, yes, the appearance, elasticity, and feel of the skin will change, but we are not talking about facial beauty. As far as the function and appearance of your body is concerned, it's all about muscle.

This CANNOT BE UNDERRATED!!! If you are a woman (or guy for that matter) and you want to have the body of a 20 year old when you are 50, you simply MUST stop thinking of working out in terms of how much cardio you can fit in! Not that keeping your heart healthy isn't important. It is, but the time you should spend on the exercycle is actually pretty small compared to how much time you many spend on it while trying to use it as the core of your program.

That is the big take home point here: if you stop making cardio the core of your fitness program you will not only be able to fundamentally change how you think of your body as you age, but you will be able to drastically reduce the TIME you spend in the gym! Instead of adding more cardio every year to keep up with your declining metabolism, you'll spend three or four hours in the gym every week, and you'll never need to increase that time expenditure, and you'll never have lie to yourself by saying "I'm working out like crazy and I'm still getting flabby, it must just be age."

Points You MUST understand:
- Just because you went to the gym doesn't mean you worked out. In fact, just because you worked up a sweat, or burned 500 calories, doesn't mean you got the kind of workout that is really investing in your anti-aging future.
- Doing a cardio class with 6 inch steps, pink 5lb dumbbells and a spunky instructor, may be "fun" but it isn't the most effective use of your time in the gym.
- Reconstructing cardio classes so they "look" like weight training does not make them as effective as true weight training.

- Going into the "Free Weight" section of the gym does not have to be as intimidating as it seems.

Enjoying your Workout vs. Making Progress

I cannot count the number of times I've heard this "I just love the new exercise program I've started. It's so much fun!" While enjoying your workout is a big deal, what good is enjoying it if it's not effective???

You absolutely must evaluate the workouts you are doing based on the fundamental principles we will discuss later. If you do not, then no matter how fun the workout is, to some extent you will be wasting your time.

If you can do your "fun" cardio class with enough intensity then you will have accomplished the cardio part of your fitness program (although less time efficiently than just doing intervals), but don't let that be an excuse for skipping the stuff that's really going to keep you young.

Free Weight Section Shouldn't be Intimidating

The first thing you need to realize is that many of those guys in the free weight section do not have a clue what they are doing. If you are a tiny female, an old man, or completely out of

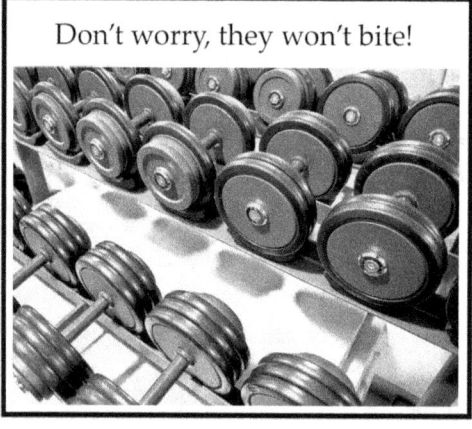

Don't worry, they won't bite!

shape and you've read this book, chances are those of us who know what we're doing are going to have the GREATEST respect for you when you walk into the free weight section. The second you pick up a couple of dumbbells and start doing Elevated Split Squats, One Arm Rows, Stiff Leg Deadlifts, or proper Military Presses, there's not going to be anyone there that has anything but respect for you.

Yes, I know, if you're an even reasonably attractive female, you're probably going to get hit on, but that happens even in the grocery store or at the gas pump and it doesn't stop you from eating or filling up your car, does it?

Here's how to make the transition from cardio class or machines into the free weight section:

- Write your workout down ahead of time. Know the exercises you want to do.
- Practice your form at home without weights.
- Scout out the free weight section first. Figure out where everything is so that you are more confident and not just wandering around looking for where everything is.
- If you don't want attention, put on some loose clothing that is comfortable but covers you up. (this is true for you guys with your 13in arms walking in with your muscle shirts as well).
- Get yourself an MP3 player with some music that is motivating. It will help block out distractions and will go a long way from keeping other people from bothering you.
- Make your first trip short and easy. Work up to the long intense workouts over time.

There you go, now put down those pink dumbbells and get ready to look fit and attractive wayyy sooner than you ever thought possible.

Stop Thinking about Calories!!

As long as you continue to think of exercise as a way of burning calories, or of eating in terms of how many calories are in something, you will always struggle with your weight!

This is an advanced philosophical concept, but an important one for long term success. For many of you, this will appear to be counter intuitive and in all probability, until you get to a fairly advanced level it will not make sense. But do not worry about it not making sense yet! Put it in the back of your brain and come back to it later. As with everything else in this book, don't let it get you down if you still have a ways to go. As I said earlier, whether it takes months or years, it WILL be a journey worth taking.

Weight loss is easily the number one fitness goal, and for good reason. It's true that all else being equal, how many calories you burn, and how many calories you consume are really what will determine how much weight you lose or gain (despite what the commercials will try to tell you).

So how can I tell you that you will eventually need to stop thinking in terms of calories? Because, almost without exception, almost every truly fit person I've ever known, doesn't think in those terms. I know this is EXTREMELY difficult for many people to grasp, as calories have been the be-all-end-all of weight maintenance for so long.

Calorie Consumption

Let's start with calorie consumption. Although at the start, you will want to monitor your calorie intake, but as you progress, you'll quickly find that there are many high calorie foods that are very healthy, and that fill you up and don't seem to hurt your waistline, and there are a lot of low calorie foods that will do the opposite.

At the beginning, your body weight may be a predominant factor in your overall health, but in the long run, you'll find you're better off thinking in terms of "Is this healthy?" or "Should I be eating this at this time of day?" and not "How many calories are in this?" Don't worry too much about this part of the calorie equation though. Not worrying about the calories in the food you eat will come naturally with time.

Know the Real Reason for Your Workout

A more important factor than not worrying about the calories you eat, and the one that many find extremely hard to master is that you absolutely MUST stop thinking in terms of "how many calories did my workout burn?"

Why? First, because you can out-eat ANY workout program. Don't believe me? Attend any marathon or better yet, an Ironman Triathlon. Look at all the chubby, overweight, and sometimes even obese individuals among the amateur competitors. Here are a group of individuals who simply in order to compete in the event, had to have been doing at least 10-15 hours of cardio PER WEEK!!

I am not saying cardio, or working out in general is not a part of your weight loss or maintenance plan, but psychologically, if you are dependent on "doing a little extra cardio tomorrow" to make up for the bad meal you had tonight, you're on the wrong track.

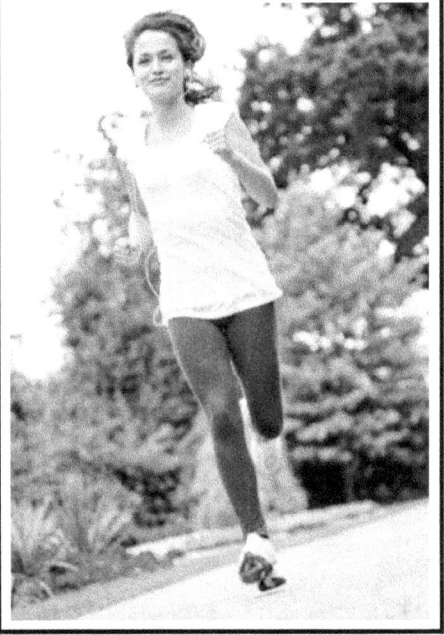

I'm NOT saying going for a run on a beautiful day is a bad thing. Just do it because you enjoy it, NOT because it's burning off the cheat meal the night before!

Your weight loss or maintenance goals absolutely MUST be centered on a proper nutrition plan. However, your workout program must be based on goals other than how many calories they burn. Your reason for a specific workout may be to put on muscle (so you can burn more calories long term) or increase your aerobic threshold, but just burning calories cannot be the reason for going to the gym or getting on the treadmill.

In fact, many experienced fitness enthusiasts like myself, will actually LOSE weight if we are forced to not workout for some period of time, mainly because we are so aware of our own bodies, that without even thinking about it, we will back off on the food intake.

I have found that for just about anyone I've ever worked with, it is simply too difficult to maintain long term motivation for working out based on the ability of the workouts to burn calories. If you can maintain long term motivation based on burning calories, your workouts will reflect this, and you'll end up being that "skinny fat" person who can't figure out why they're aging despite 10 hours a week in the gym.

Yes, you will burn off a couple cookies with an hour on the treadmill, but you can add enough extra muscle through weight training that you may never have to worry about excess body fat. But regardless of the type of workout you are doing, if burning some calories is the goal of the workout, you will be much more likely to NOT make it to the gym than if your goal is more tangible.

Better Reasons For Your Workout

What do I mean by tangible? Adding some muscle so that you have that strong "toned" look, or pushing out some serious intervals on the treadmill so that your cardio capacity is where it needs to be for your lifestyle (running that marathon, playing ball with the younger guys at work, or just keeping up with your kids).

Why isn't weight loss tangible? Because it's just not an efficient way of losing weight, and eventually you will figure that out and lose motivation.

You will absolutely find you are more motivated long term if these are the sort of reasons you have for getting into the gym. As you start to learn just how much time you have to spend in the gym to burn off one bad dietary mistake, you will realize these types of goals are much more concrete.

Also, because you no longer think in terms of making up for bad dietary decisions with extra time in the gym, you will be less likely to make those bad decisions in the first place.

46

The efficiency of your overall program will improve as well. Once you adopt this way of thinking, you'll no longer even think of just hopping on the elliptical for 45 minutes "for some cardio." Cardio time will become "time to work on my anaerobic threshold," or some other goal that will actually push you to new levels of fitness, and in the end, will actually end up burning even more calories in a shorter time.

In this respect, this topic mimics my earlier discussion on goals. If you just go into the gym "to get a workout," you will not be using your time most efficiently. The same is true with "burning calories." If you're just plodding along in the "cardio zone," your overall fitness will quickly cease to improve, and you really won't be burning a lot of calories.

At some point, this transition to a new way of thinking will occur naturally, as long as you're following the other advice in this book. Weight control will no longer be an issue for you, as your diet will be clean (most of the time), and your workouts will be of sufficient intensity, that your metabolism will be high enough to burn off any cheat meals you choose to have.

But I still advise you to try to make this transition in the way you think about exercise as soon as possible. Have a goal for each and every workout that involves improving some aspect of your fitness level. Never say, "I can eat this tonight because I'm going to do an extra hour of cardio tomorrow," and you'll soon find yourself graduating to a level of self awareness that you'll need if you want to stay fit for the rest of your life.

How Your Body Adapts

Here's a concept that should be a little easier to grasp than the last one, and may help reinforce it a little: Your fitness improves as a result of your workouts (after your workouts), not during them.

Of the following two examples of this, one is pretty well known while the other isn't brought up very often.

Pretty much everyone knows that you don't get stronger or bigger WHILE you're lifting weights. In fact we even use statements like "I really destroyed my legs today," to describe a good workout. We know that we may very well be damaging the very muscle tissue we are trying to build. Your body will say to itself "What's going on here? Looks like our lifestyle has changed and we can't afford to be fat and weak anymore. We better build some muscle." Of course your body doesn't really talk to itself, but the feedback mechanisms that your body uses to adapt are every bit as complex, if not more so, than any decision you can make consciously.

Here's an example that isn't so widely discussed but just as real: If you're doing a lot of cardio in the "fat burning zone" you are signaling your body to store as much fat as efficiently as possible. Your body is saying to itself (hypothetically) "Wow, we're sure doing a lot of activity that requires fat for energy and doesn't really strain our muscles at all. I better get rid of all this excess muscle, and store as much fat as possible."

Yes, it really does work like this. It's why you'll see so many people struggling with their bodyweight despite tons of cardio. It's also why you'll always see all the flabby people in the cardio classes or laboring away on the elliptical, and all the really fit people in the free weight room or out sprinting or climbing stairs at the local high school track.

Of course, there are many other fitness related parameters our bodies can adapt to. Your nervous system doesn't get more efficient allowing you to become stronger, until you rest and let it adapt. You don't add more mitochondria and supportive tissue that allows your muscles to do more work for longer, until you rest, etc., etc.

What can we learn from this? We learn that doing steady state cardio in the "fat burning zone" is a sure way to signal our bodies to try their hardest to store more body fat and lose muscle in preparation for future steady state cardio (more on the better way to do cardio later).

We also can deduce that for most goals, adequate rest is just as important as the workout. There's no sure rule for how much rest you need for a given workout, that's something you will have to learn about yourself, but if you're not even thinking in those terms, you will certainly never figure it out.

We'll talk more about stress in the next chapter, but we can also deduce from the above information that if the body needs to recover from our workouts, it probably also needs to recover from any other stressor, and if your body has multiple stressors to recover from, it's going to take more time to recover.

So there you have it, some philosophical stuff to roll around in your head. No, I'm not trying to turn health and fitness into some kind of religion by trying to force you to think the way I think. But from experience, I know that if you come to terms with the above topics, you will have a much easier time on your road to lifelong fitness.

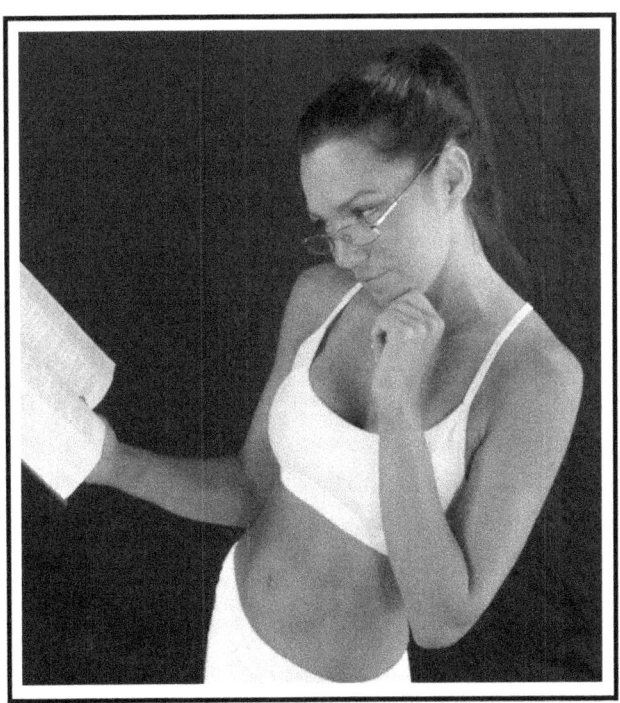

Chapter 3 – It's all in the details

This chapter will deal with a number of details that won't specifically be about working out or nutrition, but will be very useful if you're really serious about understanding how to create a fitness program that is right for you.

How much time will my goal take?

"Abs of Steel in only 5 minutes a day!!!?!!" If any of you still believe this article, then either you're eternally optimistic, or you've never bothered to try and get in shape. While the vast majority of the fitness industry tries to sell you on the concept that fitness is easy and quick (as long as you buy their gadget, gimmick, or pill), I earn my living with an honest, realistic approach to fitness (How silly of me!).

I realize that many people have trouble putting their workout time into perspective. I frequently get asked "How much time do I have to spend in the gym to look like you?" or "How much time do you think she spends in the gym?" This section is in hopes of providing some realistic estimates.

How am I coming up with the estimates I'm going to provide? Quite frankly, through personal experience alone. I have no studies to back me up, I'm just using my years in the business, and the hundreds of clients I've worked with and made a lot of assumptions. Also, remember that genetics play a BIG role in all of this. Some people can make a lot of progress with less effort, but this doesn't take away from the general validity of my estimates for the average person reading this.

First, let's start by looking at how many hours you have in a week: 168. Of that most of you spend 48 of that sleeping (should be closer to 60 for optimum health and mental alertness), 21 eating, and 45 working and commuting. That leaves 54 hours a week for everything else including working out.

You can subtract from that number for your particular situation, but please be honest with yourself. If you put 30 hours for taking care of the kids, but 15 of that is all of you sitting in front of the TV, then maybe you need to reevaluate more than just your workouts.

I've noticed that the people who actually have the most time constraints are the ones who complain about them the least. I would have a single mom working two jobs AND taking care of the kids, who would always find the time to workout. Many gyms have free daycare, and I'm told by my clients who are parents that their kids absolutely love going, and even help motivate them to get to the gym!

On one occasion, I had an elderly female client. She was only with us for two months, but in that time she made incredible progress. Her quality of life improved dramatically. Her family was ecstatic! I was assured by her husband and children that money was not a problem, and that the improvements in her mobility and energy level were almost miraculous.

Her reason for quitting? She didn't have the time! Now realize, she was long retired, her kids were out of the house, and as far as anyone could tell, she didn't have a single real obligation that could possibly be more important than her health. What was her real reason for quitting? I could probably take a guess, but I'll really never know.

Just realize that your excuse that you don't have enough time, really is just an excuse. Now for some estimates:

**ALERT – The following estimates ASSUME you are doing QUALITY workouts. Sitting on the exercycle with the pedals barely moving does not qualify as a cardio workout, and doing 5lb dumbbell curls is not a resistance workout!

General Health

Let's start with general health. Let's say you're not overweight, but have a non-active lifestyle, and you just want to stay reasonably healthy. You'd like to minimize your chances of

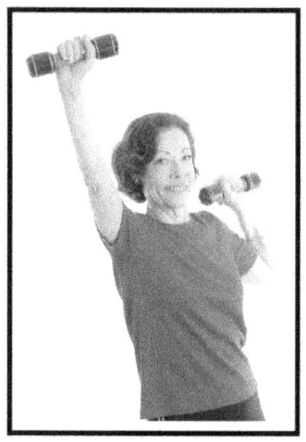

having a heart attack or back problems, and you'd like to age gracefully without ending up in a wheelchair long before your time is up. This will also assume you do not have to lose any weight and that your diet is otherwise healthy.

Believe it or not, you can probably do this in as little as two and a half hours a week. My recommendations are two 30-minute resistance-training sessions with stretching along with three 30-minute sessions of cardio. These workouts should be divided up throughout the week, and you should be exerting yourself even if you don't get anywhere close to over exerting yourself (you should feel tired but still energetic and able to go on with your day after your workouts). If you'd like to divide these workouts up into smaller, more frequent workouts that you can do without needing a shower afterwards, you can probably count on upping the total to three hours per week, but at less intensity.

This is actually quite amazing given that our ancestors were active for almost the entire waking day. The fact that we can stay healthy with such a small amount of activity is pretty amazing. I do recommend more activity than that. Even something as insignificant as parking at the far end of a parking lot or taking the stairs instead of the elevator, can all really add up when you are working towards general health.

Remember, the proceeding advice is no guarantee of good health. You can do everything right and still get cancer, just as some people can do everything wrong and live to be 100.

Weight Loss

What if you're trying to lose weight? Well of course you can do what a lot of people do and just starve yourself, but then you'll end up lighter, not much healthier, and you'll have lost up to half of that weight in muscle instead of fat. You will still look flabby, and you'll probably feel terrible. You'll also probably gain it all back rather quickly.

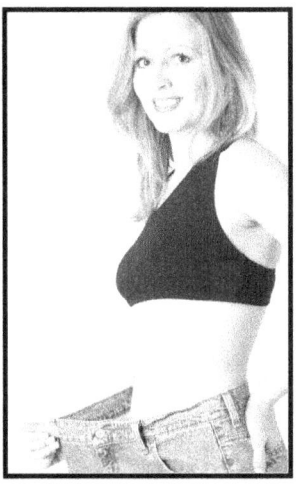

If you want to lose weight the healthy way, and end up looking thin AND firm, you'll want to count on doing about four and a half hours per week of vigorous exercise along with a healthy (but not starvation) diet. I recommend three 45 minute resistance training sessions every week to prevent muscle loss (due to calorie reduction), and speed up the metabolism all day long, and three 45 minute cardio sessions to keep the heart healthy and burn extra calories. Don't try to make up for a bad diet with extra cardio. It will take an extra hour on the treadmill to make up for a couple of cookies. Be realistic. With this time commitment you may look for a pound of healthy fat loss per week - if you're doing everything right.

Beach Fit

Now what if you've slimmed down but want a body that looks good in a bathing suit? You don't want to be a fitness model, but you'd like to be proud of what you've got. Maybe you're getting into your forties, and want to look like you did when you were in your twenties. For this goal, four and a half hours will also usually do the trick. Except in this case you'll change the split between resistance training and cardio. An hour and a half of cardio each week will be enough to keep your heart healthy. Three twenty minute sessions every week may even be enough, as long as they are interval workouts.

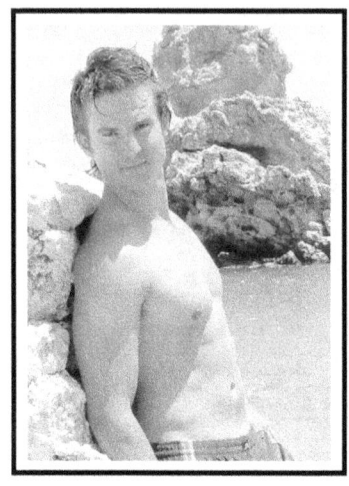

In fact, I know many who have very fit and trim bodies that do almost nothing that resembles traditional cardio, and instead get all of their heart health from fast-paced resistance training sessions. As with much of the advice in this book, this will vary from individual to individual.

For this goal of really looking firm and toned, you'll need to up the amount of time with the weights. I'd recommend four 45 minute sessions every week. For both men and women, firm, toned muscle is really what will make you look good in a bathing suit (to combat the muscle you'd normally lose as you age).

Fabulously Fit

Now what if you want a truly phenomenal physique - the kind of body that could almost be on the cover of a fitness magazine. The kind of body that doesn't just get looks at the

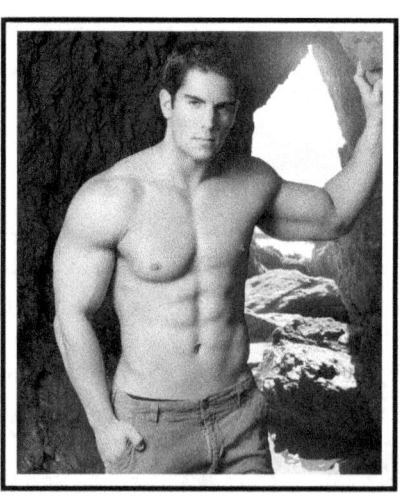

beach, it gets envious stares! With the exception of very young females with surgical augmentation, everyone I've ever met or worked with that got to this point put somewhere on the order of six to ten hours a week into working out!

Usually you'll need five or six sessions of resistance training per week, and the remainder as high intensity cardio and sports. Frequently, most of the cardio comes from some sort of enjoyable sport, since very few people can keep up this sort of routine day after day in a gym without burning out. If you do enjoy your gym workouts enough to not need enjoyable sporting activities, you may end up closer to the six hour per week figure, as high intensity gym workouts will usually be more time efficient than sporting activities, although not as enjoyable for most people.

I've observed that these types of people rarely miss a workout, and when they are in the gym or on the playing field, they hit it with an intensity that will draw stares from others nearby. Their diets are usually meticulous enough that their friends are always making fun of the food they eat.

I'm going to stop there. I won't even bother to talk about athletes or bodybuilders. Those fields are beyond my scope, and most will frequently dedicate most of their lives to workouts of some sort. Neither athletes nor bodybuilders are any more "healthy" than the other categories above, nor will they necessarily appear more fit and attractive. They will simply be better at their sport.

Me

So many people ask how much I work out that I think it may be a helpful addition here. As a little background for those

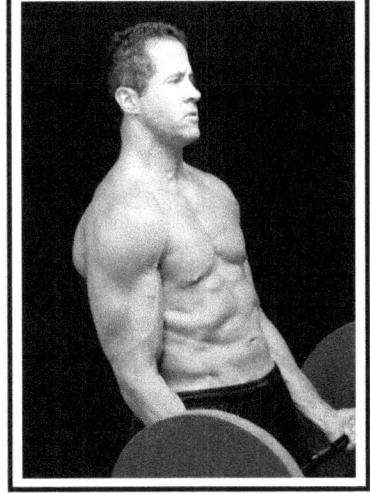

who have never met me, I am in my 40's, 6'1" and generally run a little under 200 lbs at about 9% body fat. This picture is me, but after a couple of months of really stepping up the diet and workouts. I'm about 6% body fat there and about 193lbs. I get looks on the beach regardless of whether I'm in "photo shoot" shape or not, and in fact, many people say I look better overall at 9% body fat. I do NOT have excellent genetics (See my picture earlier in the book), and struggled with my weight for the first half of my life. Adding muscle was always a battle because when I ate enough to add muscle, the body fat would come back as well.

My normal routine usually takes up about four and a half hours per week, not including any sports I may be participating in. I will generally do five or six 45 minute sessions per week. I will generally work my cardio (almost strictly time efficient intervals that I'll get into later) in with my normal workout, so sometimes a workout may only take 35 minutes and sometimes 55, depending on how many intervals I do, or what type of resistance training session.

I'm probably on the far end of the cardio spectrum, and find that I generally look my best with minimum cardio to distract from my resistance training. During the winter months, I usually have to force myself to do a couple interval sessions every week just to make sure I'm not sucking wind on the mountain bike come springtime.

I keep a pretty clean diet 90% of the time, but I do cheat with the occasional ice cream cone, pint of beer or plate of fries. As with many things, how you would view my diet depends largely on your perspective. People who don't know me well (and don't see me at home), think it's unfair that I can stay as fit as I am and eat the stuff I eat, but my girlfriend will tell you just how frustratingly clean my diet is as she sees what I really eat day to day.

When I want to step it up (photo shoot, vacation to the beach, etc.) and really want that six pack, then I will step it up a little in the gym, although not much. I will make sure to get in six times a week, and make sure to get the intervals in, but for the most part, the big change comes in the number of calories I consume and the type of workouts I do (www.thinkingpersonsfitness.com for my "get in shape for summer" workout).

So there you have it, 2.5hrs per week to be healthy, 4.5hrs per week for healthy weight loss or to look good, or 6-10 hours to be phenomenally fit.

Wow, up to ten hours a week working out? I guess we can all give up on having that "phenomenal physique"! I'm sure this next statistic doesn't apply to any of you, but the average American spends 20 hours per week watching TV![1] So instead of being overweight or even obese, the average American could have a phenomenal physique just by trading half the time they spend watching TV for working out. Makes you think, doesn't it!

Metabolic Rate

One question that is very important to many of the discussions in this book is: How is BMR (base metabolic rate) affected by muscle mass? BMR or RMR (resting metabolic rate) is the rate at which your body burns calories when you're doing nothing at all.

It has always been generally accepted as fact that muscle burns calories even while resting. For many years, I have seen references to the fact that each pound of muscle burns about 20 calories a day. However, if you do any searching on the internet recently, you will uncover references that state that a pound of muscle will only burn 4 extra calories per day, a pretty small amount. They will all quote the same reference.

I can only assume these authors are Richard Simmons fanatics that are upset at how low their testosterone has plummeted from doing too much cardio and wearing pink shorts. It didn't take me long to find out how incorrect they were. They had picked out a little bit of theory that supported their point of view, and ignored any other evidence to the contrary.

To get to the answer, I need to explain some theory on BMR. For many years (going back almost a century) scientists have been looking for a formula to predict BMR. Most have been based on Body Mass, Height, Age and Gender. Variations of this basic formula have existed since 1919. However, the formula has had to be revised over the years due to some unknown factor that was changing. The basics of the human body haven't changed in the last 100 years, but what has changed is the amount of muscle the average person has (due to our currently inactive lifestyles.)

Recently, a new formula was derived. This new formula is more accurate for individuals of all types, and is also simpler: It has only one variable LBM (Lean Body Mass = Muscle).

$$BMR = 370 + (21.6*LBM)$$

Where LBM = (1-Body Fat percent)*(Body Mass in Kg)

You may not care much for the math, and may never even care to calculate your BMR, but there are some interesting conclusions we can come to based on the data that generated this formula:

Bottom Line

First, short of very rare diseases, your BMR is almost entirely determined by how much muscle you have. The fact that there is only one factor relevant enough to be included in this formula shows us this. The previous, less accurate formulas used weight, height, age, and gender as a makeshift way of predicting muscle mass. This is why the formula had to keep changing.

Based on the data that generated the formula, muscle uses 21.6 calories per day per pound (about what we've always thought to be the case), not 4 as quoted in the articles mentioned above, and the rest of your body accounts for about 370 calories per day regardless of how big you are or what gender.

This isn't theoretical, it's what the researchers tested in thousands of individuals. This means that in one year, one extra pound of muscle will burn over 7600 calories, or over two pounds of body fat. If you consider that the average American puts on 1-1.5lbs of fat per year, you begin to see just how significant a couple extra pounds of muscle can be for your long term weight maintenance!

Yes, adding a pound of extra muscle could completely compensate for the weight gain the average American experiences as they age!

What Doesn't Matter

The next fact we can derive from this research is that neither height, age, nor gender affect BMR. The fact that height really doesn't matter shouldn't surprise anyone. Age is also no big surprise. You'll often hear that our metabolism slows down as we age. This is not true to any great extent. Our metabolism slows down as we lose muscle, and since the average sedentary American loses muscle as they age, the metabolism slows down. I personally feel that this misrepresentation of the facts by many health care practitioners does us all a great disservice: What most American's have been told is normal, may be average, but not normal in any physiological sense.

I will repeat this as it is SOO important. If you maintain your muscle as you age, your metabolism will not slow down to any significant extent. Yes, there are factors like declining hormones which may affect metabolism to some small extent, but as far as I can find in my research, no one has yet to show any significant effect independent of muscle mass.

How about gender? I see the commercials all the time that tell women they are different from men. They don't lose weight as easily, or need pills made especially for them, etc. Although there are certainly many difference between men and women, metabolism isn't one of them. Putting on a couple extra pounds of muscle will help a woman just as much as it will help a man. The smaller amount of muscle many women start with only makes the effect more pronounced, as each pound of muscle you add will have a greater percentage effect on your metabolism.

So cheer up girls, despite what the commercials tell you, your base metabolism works the same as it does for guys.

Body Fat Percent

Body fat percent is exactly what it sounds like: the percent of your body which is made up of body fat. At any given body weight, if you have a higher body fat percent, you will have less muscle mass and therefore a slower metabolism.

How is body fat calculated? Well, the short answer is: Not very well. If you've had your body fat measured for free by the guy in the gym who is responsible for initiating new members, then you've probably had it taken extremely inaccurately.

There are several scientific methods of determining body fat percentage, including weighing you in a tank of water, and scanning you using x-rays (DEXA), but both of these methods are expensive, time consuming and out of the reach of most of us.

The most common method you will see is the use of a body fat measuring scale or device you hold in each hand that runs a small electrical current through your body, to purportedly determine your body fat level. This method is not only highly inaccurate, but also terribly bad at even establishing a trend.

The problem with this method is that it cannot distinguish between fat and muscle. If you workout, or just naturally have a little more muscle than average, the sensors will read this as fat. Very athletic individuals will typically display almost comical results. As an example, I typically measure around 9% body fat with any reasonably accurate method. In any case, just by looking at me with my shirt off, anyone with any background in fitness would immediately say I am under 10-15% without any doubt. The bio-impedance devices will typically say I am around 25% body fat. I have never had one of those devices read lower than 20%, and have had them overestimate to over 30%.

Even if you are an "average" individual, as you proceed to get in shape, lose fat, and gain muscle, the device will tell you that you are not making any progress at all. I don't know about you, but it sounds like a pretty useless device to me!

Accurately Determining BF

So how do you find an accurate body fat estimate of yourself without access to a sports science laboratory? It's actually fairly simple, but not easy. Skin Fold tests with a specialized caliper are actually very accurate IF done by a trained and experienced professional. This is actually a big IF, as most people are not properly trained or experienced. I once heard a researcher say that he wouldn't consider a testers results to be accurate until they had run the test on over 1000 people. I think this is a bit much, but the point is made: This method requires some skill to perform accurately.

If you are not sure of the experience of the individual doing the test for you, here are some things to look out for. First, if they try to give you results based on a single test of a single part of your body, RUN, don't walk, to someone else who has a clue. There are formulas which are reasonable with a three site test, but formulas which use five or more sites are even better. If the tester is good enough at it to take their results seriously, they should be able to take the same measurements again (without looking at what they did the first time) and get essentially identical results.

Next, make sure if you will be getting before and after tests, that you have the same person do the testing and use the same sites and techniques. Keep all of your before measurements (not just the resulting body fat percent), so that you can compare the individual site measurements for anything that might look inconsistent (ex. Four of your sites go down and one goes up drastically).

If done properly and consistently, having your body fat measured is not only the best way to determine your BMR, but also a good way to keep accurate track of your progress (much better than the scale).

What Does the Number Look Like?

Let's look at a couple of specific examples, but before we do, we need to have some perspective on what various body fat percentages look like on both men and women. These are VERY general, and there are always exceptions to these guidelines, but the trends are still there.

At 25% body fat and above a man is considered "Obese."[2] This is certainly not scientific, but in today's society, most people won't notice a guy to be obviously overweight until above about 18%, and I have found that a man can generally look "fit" with his clothes on up to about 15% body fat. In a bathing suit, a guy will have no real noticeable body fat at about 11%. At 9% most men will start to have distinct abs, and by 6% guys will be "ripped" with a very defined six pack, veins, and lots of visible muscle definition. Most men will have a hard time maintaining a body fat level below 10%, as the body will start to rebel, lowering your thyroid output, and increasing your hunger level.

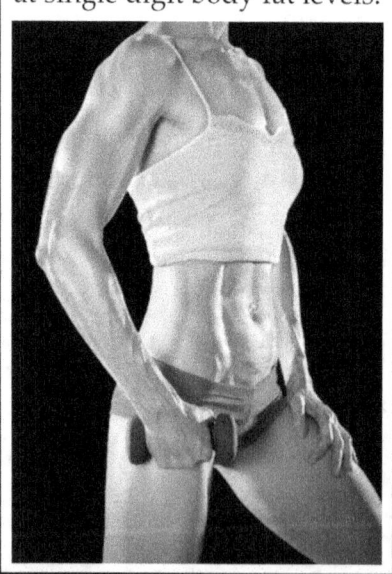

Beauty is in the eye of the beholder, but a woman's body will start to shut down at single digit body fat levels.

Women will have a higher body fat level for almost all levels of fitness, and also will look "attractive" with a much broader range of body fat levels. Although a female is considered obese at 30% body fat, I've seen examples of women generally considered to be attractive up to almost 23% body fat. Most people will start to comment on how "fit" a woman is at around 18% body fat or lower (as long as the muscle is there as well of course). Competitive fitness and bikini competitors can look attractive and feminine down to about 8-10% body fat, but at that level many people outside of the fitness world would consider them much too "ripped". At around 12% body fat, most women start to lose their period, as their body no longer considers itself healthy enough for childbirth.

How Does it Affect your BMR?

Let's see some examples of how body fat percentage can affect your base or resting metabolic rate:

We'll start with a 200 lb man. First, an average American with 22% body fat. Running through the calculations gives us a BMR of 1900 calories per day. Next is this same man once he loses some body fat and puts on some muscle. At the same weight as before, but with 10% body fat, this man has a BMR of 2140 calories per day. That's an extra 240 calories burned every day, day in and day out. That's 87,600 calories per year!! The equivalent of 146 hours on the treadmill. All without doing anything extra!

Another example: How about two women, both who are 45 years old and were a fit 130 lbs in their early twenties. The first one maintains her body weight through diet and cardio alone, and at 45, although she still weighs 130 lbs, she has lost 10 pounds of lean muscle over the years (a half pound per year is about the average muscle loss as sedentary women age).

The second woman has maintained her weight through a combination of proper nutrition, reasonable cardio and a consistent resistance training program. She is not only the same weight she was in her early twenties, looks pretty much just as fit, but she also has a BMR 210 calories per day higher than the first woman. And, as if that weren't bad enough, from this point forward, the first women will need to spend an extra 153 hours a year on the treadmill to maintain her weight. This is above and beyond what she had to do to maintain her weight when she was in her twenties, whereas woman number two can just keep doing what she's been doing all along.

I've noticed some people start to feel dejected and hopeless during discussions of body fat. Please don't let it get you down. It's just knowledge, and in the end, if you were the type of person who thought that "ignorance is bliss" you probably wouldn't be reading this book in the first place. Just take it for what it is and move on.

Calories Per Day?

BMR is just part of the energy we burn on a daily basis. Some people like to plan their calorie intake based on an assumed number of calories used. If you want to finish calculating how many calories you burn on a daily basis, you have to multiply your BMR by your activity multiplier:[3]

- Sedentary = BMR X 1.2 (little or no exercise, desk job)
- Lightly Active = BMR X 1.375 (light exercise/sports 1-3 days/wk)
- Moderately Active = BMR X 1.55 (moderate exercise/sports 3-5 days/wk)
- Very Active = BMR X 1.725 (hard exercise/sports 6-7 days/wk)
- Extra Active = BMR X 1.9 (hard daily exercise/sports & physical job or 2X day training, i.e. marathon, contest etc.)

Once you have your total calories calculated, you can subtract some number of calories (say 500 for a 1lb a week weight loss) and get your desired calories per day.

Of course, this factor introduces a large amount of error into the equation. Let's say your BMR is 1500 cal/day and you use the "Moderately Active" factor when you're really "Lightly Active". That error would introduce a calorie error of 260 calories/day, which would be enough to cause you to lose far less weight than you thought you should, but at least it's a starting point.

You can use this information to calculate how many calories you're using, and then adjust your food intake accordingly. Just remember, it's REALLY easy to fool yourself. A little fudging here and there, and the calculation is worthless. Ultimately, the best way to adjust your daily calorie intake is by monitoring your body fat or at least your weight loss (or gain if you're trying to put on muscle), and adjusting accordingly. The real usefulness of this information is more in how it helps you understand how your body is using calories.

Body Mass Index

While we're on the subject, let's talk briefly about BMI. BMI is Body Mass Index, and it's a statistic that has absolutely no use or relevance outside of research on large populations.

If you see or hear an individual or organization using BMI as it applies to an individual, do not listen to another word they say, as they are obviously completely clueless (no, I'm really not being overly dramatic).

BMI is defined as:

$$BMI = \frac{mass(lb) \times 4.88}{height^2(ft^2)}$$

BMI was invented as a research tool. It was meant to allow studies to classify large groups of individuals. Since it is so terribly limited in the information it can provide, it was never meant to be used on individuals.

Why is it so bad? Because by attempting to classify someone by their height and weight only, regardless of body fat percentage, you end up with a pretty irrelevant statistic.

If you are at all athletic, and had some ignorant health care practitioner tell you to go on a diet because you're obese (at 9% BF), you'll understand just what I mean. Yes, according to this statistic, I and many other very fit individuals are borderline obese or actually obese.

The fact that a nurse or physician could be that blindly ignorant is a topic for another book entirely.

Why is it useful when studying large groups of people? Because at that point you just don't have any more data, and you are just hoping non-average people like me cancel themselves out (when averaged in with those who have less than average muscle mass). Yes, the data probably gets a little cloudy, but at least it's something, and as long as they don't draw any exact conclusions, the study can still be relevant.

Stress

The next couple of sections in this chapter are venturing even further from what many of you expected to read about, but they are all relevant topics, that I get asked about all the time. Don't fall asleep on me yet.

Although it may seem to be a little unrelated to exercise or fitness, stress and fitness are actually very related. Exercise in and of itself is a stressor (something that causes stress). Whether it's cardio capacity or building muscle, your body responds to the stress you put on it during exercise by forcing itself to adapt so that it can better deal with the stress the next time around.

When you are over-stressed due to work or home life, the stresses will add up, and your body will not be able to deal with them all at once. Long before research showed a link between what we think and how our bodies react, our ancestors intuitively knew that our bodies could be negatively affected by too much stress.

The immune system is probably the first to be affected. Studies show that the stress put on our bodies from exercise is good for our immune systems only up to a certain point. At some point the cumulative stress of both the workouts and life itself will cause our immune system to lower its response to diseases.

Even if you don't get sick because you are over stressing your body, you will find that your workouts will drop in effectiveness. Personally, my body agrees. I find it nearly impossible to make any progress in the gym during times in my life when I'm overstressed.

Some stress is good. Just as with working out, taking all stress out of life will allow the body to de-adapt. Isolating yourself from all of life's little annoyances will not help your brain any more than sitting on the couch all day will help your body. You need some stress. The key is how much.

That's an answer you'll need to find for yourself. As with so much else in this book, it will vary greatly from individual to individual. I know some things that would stress many people out completely, don't bother me at all, but other things that would seem minor to most people will really stress me out.

It really is a balance you need to learn for yourself, and it is an important balance for far more reasons than I can go into here. Just realize, as far as exercise and fitness goals are concerned, what's going on in the rest of your life really can greatly affect your progress in the gym.

Some ways to control stress:[4]

- Identify areas of stress.
- Seek support from family and friends
- Meditation and prayer have been shown to help reduce stress levels.
- Schedule quiet times around meals. Eating while stressed may be twice as bad for you.
- Look into support groups for stress areas that can't be eliminated (divorce, death of a loved one, etc.).
- Use your stress to make you more productive when it helps (get you ramped up for a big presentation, for instance), then let go of it when it is not useful (meditation or prayer before bed time).
- Get plenty of sleep (most adults function best on 8 to 9 hours per night).
- Stay active. Some form of regular exercise will help you keep stress under control, as long as you're not overdoing it at those tough times in your life.

Of course, one of the most common methods of dealing with stress is through various prescription drugs or alcohol. I'll talk more about alcohol later, and prescription drugs are beyond my area of expertise, but always remember, there's no free lunch. Relying on long term use of drugs for almost any reason has a price. If you do have a stressful time in your life and prescription drugs appear to be a good answer, make sure you are getting advice from an expert (psychiatrist, physician). Don't take this lightly. I'm sure we all know someone who has been addicted to mood altering drugs. Certainly, any drugs I know of that help with stress will quite possibly affect weight gain and many will negatively affect your workouts.

Surgery

Ok, I'll start by saying I'm not a surgeon, and have never worked in the industry, so any advice I give here is from a fitness professional who is not only well read on the subjects, but also has firsthand experience with literally hundreds of people who have undergone either bariatric or cosmetic surgery.

Why am I including it in this book? Because so many of you are working out to either look better, lose weight, or both. Many times my clients have viewed surgery as a replacement for proper nutrition and exercise, and when they do, it NEVER works out the way they had hoped!!

We'll start with cosmetic surgery. Cosmetic surgery is obviously a very broad topic. Only two types of cosmetic surgery are really relevant here: Liposuction, and skin removal/tightening. I won't spend time going into the various dangers and complications of each procedure. Most seem to be reasonably safe, with the majority of complications coming from a relative few individual surgeons.

As with any surgery, shop carefully for a surgeon. Not only are you quite possibly putting your life on the line, but I've also seen drastically different results depending on the surgeon.

Make sure you have seen plenty of examples of your surgeons work, and that you really like the results.

Liposuction

I'm sure I don't need to tell everyone what these surgeries are, but starting with liposuction, which is the process of removing fat cells from in between the skin and underlying organs and muscle tissue. There are various techniques, and each surgeon seems to have a specific technique they prefer.

Most surgeons will tell you the same thing I'm about to. Lipo is intended for removal of stubborn fat deposits from someone who is otherwise happy with the rest of their body. If you are overweight and you have more than one or two trouble spots, exercise will do a much better job. If you do a search on the Internet, one sentiment you will see over and over is that liposuction is a body shaping procedure, not a means of weight loss.

There are two problems with using lipo to remove more than small trouble areas. The first and most important is the increased risk of surgical complications when large amounts of fat are removed. I won't go into all the complications that are possible during a surgery of this type (you can find this info on the Internet as well as from your surgeon), but the consensus seems to be that a removal of more than 8lbs of fat will greatly increase the possibility of complications. Remember, this procedure is destructively removing living tissue from your body! The blood loss and tissue damage can be extensive!

The second issue with liposuction is that the area where the fat is removed may be smaller, but will sometimes look lumpy or deformed. Using a good surgeon will certainly help here, but the more fat that is removed, the more likely that the affected area will not look aesthetically pleasing. I feel that results are generally much more appealing if less than 4lbs need to be removed

I think liposuction can be a really great option for people who have worked hard to get into shape, are maintaining a good diet and exercise program, but have a problem location that just doesn't want to change. Often, a client will get to a point where they love the way their entire body looks except for one spot. They'll try to lose a little more weight, and that may help that one spot but then the rest of their body starts looking too thin. Friends tell them their face looks drawn, and they start looking older as a result.

I can completely understand how someone can let that one problem spot drive them crazy after all that hard work in the gym. Liposuction may be their only option to ever be satisfied with their body.

The problem I have with liposuction is that a majority of liposuction is performed on individuals who still have significant weight to lose. They may say they only have one problem area, but then after the first surgery, they see another area that annoys them, then another, and another.

Over the years, I have seen dozens of examples of people who no longer looked like real people. They had several (in some cases dozens) of operations, and the fat distribution was grotesquely disproportionate. Maybe they had a thin waist, thighs and butt, but with flabby arms, big ankles, double chins, and lumpy and badly distributed fat even in the areas of surgery.

Even the best surgeon cannot make the results look natural if they take too much fat out. I will honestly say that I find an overweight person more aesthetically pleasing than many of the people I have seen who go crazy with the liposuction.

Even if you don't go crazy, many people who don't get to their target weight before having surgery, just end up being dissatisfied with another area of their body. This is a personal observation only, and I don't have any facts to back it up, but I would say 90% of the people I have known to get lipo would have been much happier just losing a little more weight.

Another problem is that if you don't already have your diet and exercise program in order, you will just gain the fat back elsewhere. Yes, you have fewer fat cells in that specific area of the body, and that area will always be thinner than other areas, but that doesn't stop your body from storing fat elsewhere. This is another time when I've seen lipo patients look a little "off." The body is now storing fat in all sorts of weird patterns. One of the most frequent examples of this are women who get their thighs and butt liposuctioned, then start looking very "square" as their bodies start storing fat on their midsection and arms. They start looking like a chunky guy and lose all appearance of having feminine curves.

Liposuction and Cellulite

Cellulite is a condition characterized by dimpling of the skin over fat, often referred to as "cottage cheese" skin. Cellulite is caused by fibrous bands of connective tissue that are connected to the undersurface of the skin. As you age, if you are not exercising vigorously, you lose muscle and gain body fat. This combination of effects stretches these bands of connective under the skin. Cellulite is not improved significantly by liposuction because it is not just a matter of body fat, but also muscle and the connective tissue. Liposuction may sometimes make cellulite appear worse, especially in older individuals.

The only real way to lessen the appearance of cellulite is to build up the muscle underneath the area and lower your overall body fat level; thereby allowing the bands of connective tissue to return to their normal positions.

If you are considering getting lipo, here is a checklist I would recommend you go through first.

1. Have you truly done all you can do with diet and exercise? If you once liked the way you looked, are you back to the same weight and muscle mass you had when you were happy with the way you looked? If you answered no to either of these, I would HIGHLY recommend you get that in order first. I can almost guarantee you will not be happy in the long run if you get liposuction before getting in shape.

2. Get honest opinions from people you can trust. Ask them if they agree that you only have one problem area, or would you be better off losing a little weight everywhere. Be open minded to their feedback.

3. Ask your surgeon how much fat they will have to remove. If they advise much more than 4 pounds, that may also be a sign that you are better off losing some weight first. Make sure you see pictures of the surgeons work on others with your same issues.

If you have results that either reinforce or disagree with what I have said here, I would be highly interested seeing your results. Please email me some photos.

Removal of Excess Skin

Removal or tightening of the skin is something that becomes necessary when a patient has been drastically overweight for a long period of time. At that point the skin has stretched and no amount of weight loss will cause it to return to its previous size. Many previously overweight clients have horribly embarrassing skin folds as a result.

Although I have never heard of any health risks due to this excess skin, after all that hard work losing the weight, many people just cannot tolerate it, and find it embarrassing. I cannot give you many recommendations other than to choose your surgeon wisely. From what I have seen, this surgery always results in scars. It's not a perfect option, but if it's something you want to do, I've certainly seen decent results and I've seen rather horrible results. I'm not sure how much of this depends on how much skin needs to be removed, and how much relies on the skill of the surgeon, but I would still shop around.

Bariatric Surgery

Next is bariatric surgery. Bariatric surgery is actually several different types of surgeries all which have the same goal: to limit the amount of food a patient can consume. Some do this by restricting the size of the plumbing through which the food passes, and some work by reducing the size of the stomach itself.

Proponents of bariatric surgery say it's a great way to help morbidly obese patients for whom diet and exercise have failed.

Let's be perfectly clear and blunt: Diet and exercise have never failed ANYONE. You may fail at diet and exercise, because you simply did not do what you needed to do, but diet and exercise, when done properly have never failed.

Bariatric surgery does nothing but attempt to keep someone from overeating. I say attempt, because a fairly large number of patients eventually manage to figure out more bad habits that enable them to continue to overeat.

The surgery will not make you any healthier other than helping you to lose weight. If you continue to eat calorie rich foods, and not exercise, you will still be unhealthy. The most common criteria for "success" is any case where the patient loses half their excess weight, typically 50 out of 100 lbs. The "success" rate I see most often is around 50%. In other words, the average bariatric surgery patient is still 50lbs overweight even after having this expensive and dangerous surgery.

The complications involved are also frequent and in many instances, severe. These include death during surgery (1-2.5%), hernias, blood clots, infection, failure of the surgery, gastric dumping, nutrient deficiency, gall stones, bowel disorders, etc. These complications are not rare, rather they are quite common.

These surgeries are VERY expensive ($15,000 to $30,000) and unlike cosmetic surgery, usually covered by insurance (i.e. paid for by the rest of us who have health insurance). Bariatric surgery, by definition, does nothing that simply putting down the fork and stepping away from the table couldn't do much more safely and with less of a burden on our health care system.

You won't find a lot of physicians that agree with me on this. These procedures are growing in popularity, despite the low rate of success (in my view), potential severe complications, and high cost. Of course the people who disagree with me are making a lot of money off of these procedures, and as of yet, not experiencing a major backlash of medical malpractice lawsuits, despite the high rate of serious complications. [5,6,7,89,10,11]

Massage

If you've been working out for any length of time (or simply done any manual labor, played a sport, worked in your garden, etc.) it's inevitable that you've experienced tight, sore muscles, a cramp or pulled muscle. Certainly if you experience an inordinate amount of pain, or cannot function properly, you should see your doctor immediately. However, many times sore or tight muscles are simply a consequence we live with.

Many people routinely treat muscle soreness with over the counter pain medications. What they may not realize is that although the short term discomfort is diminished, they may actually be increasing the total recovery time. You see, the inflammation that these medications are relieving are actually your body's way of healing the damaged tissue. In many instances you are just delaying the healing process. On top of this, anti-inflammatory medications such as acetaminophen (Tylenol®), ibuprofen (Advil®), and naproxen (Aleve®), can actually halt your body's recovery from all workouts. In other words, when you take those pain medications for sore quads, you've pretty much made that tough leg workout you just completed less effective.

Not that I'm saying you should throw out that bottle of Ibuprofen you have in the medicine cabinet. I'll be the first to admit that when muscle pain is keeping me from getting a good night's sleep, I'll sometimes reach for an over the counter pain reducer. But many times there is a better and even more effective way of relieving those tight, sore muscles: Massage.

I encourage all my clients to find a good deep tissue massage therapist. It's a treat you'll never regret. I've seen conflicting evidence on the ability of massage to aide in recovery from workouts, but I think that is due to bad experimental design.   No, massage will probably not help with DOMS (delayed onset muscle soreness) that a lot of us get as a typical result of a new or tougher workout, but if you really have knots or adhesions from a past injury, or a small muscle tear you never even knew you had, then I think massage can be invaluable.

I advise you to look for someone who works regularly with athletes. They will be more accustomed to the work you need done, although most therapists will be able to do what you need them to do as long as they are experienced with truly deep tissue techniques. Try a couple different therapists, and find one that you not only like but whose massage makes a distinct difference after they work on you. If not right away, at least within a day, you should feel much "looser." It's hard to describe it if you haven't felt it, but when you have a knot or serious adhesion, you will know right away when it has improved.

You'll want to be prepared for at least a little discomfort during the massage. This isn't a feel good, relaxing Swedish massage.   It's deep tissue, and will have to be a little uncomfortable to work. How uncomfortable? I've had a couple of massages that bordered on torture, and that's too deep. A good therapist should be able to go deep enough without making you so uncomfortable that you tense up. If you find yourself tensing up during the massage, then any work the therapist is doing will be for nothing. A good therapist will know this and ease up as soon as they feel you tense up, but many aren't good enough to figure that out. Find one who is. It also helps when you give them feedback as well.

Quite often the best therapist isn't the biggest guy, or the most attractive girl, or whatever your preconceived notion of a good massage therapist is. Put those prejudices aside and look for results. Many times, the best therapists may not be the busiest and may actually be more economical, just because they don't meet most people's physical expectations.

Part II – Working Out

Remember this book is not intended to be a step-by-step "how to" for getting fit. It is a series of topics that I have found to be very important to the vast majority of my clients. So, if there is a topic that you don't see, that doesn't necessarily mean I'm ignoring it, just that perhaps it's already been covered too many times elsewhere or something I just don't consider important for my typical client.

First, it's called "working" out for a reason! It should be hard work! Any device or plan that purports to make exercising "easier," is missing the point. If you are looking for the most time efficient workouts, "easy" is your enemy. In general terms, the tougher the better, whether cardio, or resistance training. Any way we can manipulate (or trick) ourselves into upping the intensity is good.

This doesn't mean jumping into a program for which you are not prepared. You will always need to ramp up the intensity gradually. If you are really out of shape and have not engaged in any significant and consistent exercise in many years, then it may take many months to up the intensity level. Don't worry about it. As long as you are always pushing yourself a little harder, the results will come.

If you think this section is a little short, then you've stumbled upon one of the secrets of the fitness industry: "This isn't rocket science." It's a secret many in the industry don't want you to discover. You see, it's hard to make money off commonly available knowledge and inexpensive free weights.

But the problem isn't that so many people are wasting their money on gadgets and gimmicks, the problem is that these gadgets, gimmicks and new programs with exotic names are distracting people from the simplest, most time efficient way of getting into shape. I've lived a pretty full life, and I've witnessed foolishness in many places, but nowhere will you see so many people thoroughly wasting their time and energy as in most commercial gyms.

You really can't blame the equipment manufacturers and fitness guru's for trying. Let's face it, every other facet of American life emphasizes "better" "faster" and "easier". How could a few dumbbells, a bench, some traditional free weight exercises, and running fast really be the best way to get in shape?

If we can make every other aspect of our lives easier, why can't we make "working out" easier as well? But therein lies the quandary. The very fact that we have taken all of the hard work out of daily life is what makes working out necessary! Ask anyone who grew up on a farm how necessary a gym was where he grew up. It wasn't.

Three quarters of a century ago, the athletes of muscle beach in California pretty much knew all they needed to know. Notice I used the word "athlete." They were not only strong, but flexible, coordinated, and fit in every sense of the word.[12] The unfortunate fact is that even though these athletes were not only capable of great feats of strength, but also incredible body weight gymnastics and flexibility demonstrations, the timid public, with the help of less than knowledgeable academics, labeled them as muscle bound freaks.

Hence was started the almost century long movement to get in shape without using the most efficient methods and equipment to do so. The aerobic craze that appeared to start in the 70's was really nothing more than an outgrowth of a century of misguided academics.

Anyone who follows politics can attest to how hard it is to be middle of the road, and hence fitness as well has seemed to be an "all or nothing" proposition. You're either a "runner," or a "bodybuilder," or you're "into yoga." It seems for most people a balanced approach to fitness is almost unimaginable.

However, that's where real fitness lies, and hence why we don't have to make this part of the book any more complicated than it needs to be.

Chapter 4 - Muscle Science

How Your Muscles Work

The science behind how your muscles work is really rather fascinating, however, as with all the other topics in this book, I'm going to simplify this subject to just the information you need to know to help you with your fitness goals.

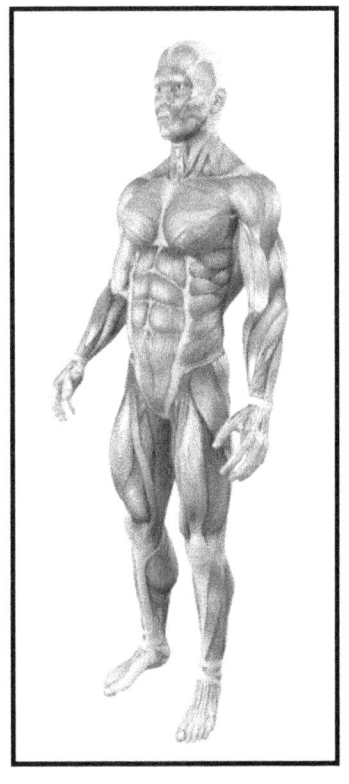

Your muscles are not much different from the muscles in a mouse or those in a whale or a bird. In fact, the individual muscle fibers are almost identical. The difference lies in the amount of each type of fiber and the way the fibers are arranged.

Fiber Type

Even within your own body, each muscle is different in the type and arrangement of the fibers. The reason for this is that each muscle has different uses, and hence different muscle fiber requirements. The most common terms you will hear are "fast twitch" and "slow twitch". Although there are more than two types of fibers, it's good enough that you understand that certain muscles have more fast twitch fibers and others have more slow twitch fibers.

A predominantly slow twitch muscle is made for slower, lower effort, longer duration movements, whereas a fast twitch fiber will be better for intense, short duration movements. Every muscle in your body has both slow and fast twitch fibers, but in different proportions. Slow twitch fibers will grow much slower than fast twitch fibers, no matter what type of training you are using, which is why some muscles seem to never grow no matter how hard you work them.

Although it is very hard to generalize, postural muscles tend to be predominantly slow twitch, while muscles such as those in your upper arms (biceps, triceps) tend to be more fast twitch.

Many people will try to base their training on the makeup of a particular muscle group: Training a predominantly fast twitch muscle with high weight, low rep sets, and training a predominantly slow twitch muscle with higher rep sets. There may be something to this, but in my mind, this is usually more complicated than it's worth.

Where I feel this knowledge comes in handy is when you realize that ANY muscle will adapt to the type of training you give it. A predominantly slow twitch muscle will transform some of the fibers into fast twitch fiber if you train it with heavy weights and fast, short sets, but is that what you really want? Sometimes, you may want a muscle that is predominantly slow twitch to get bigger and stronger. Knowing the makeup of that muscle will at least let you know that it's going to be a more difficult task.

It is also good to realize that what works for one muscle group may not work for another. Just because you can totally exhaust your arms and legs by training them heavy once or twice a week, doesn't mean that same stimulus is going to work for your calves or core, which may require more frequent stimulation.

This also holds true between different individuals. If you're workout partner is more fast twitch than you are, they are going to lift heavier and for less sets than you will need to. Other than letting someone cut into your muscles, there is no way to really know which you are, but as you train, you'll probably figure it out for yourself. Just remember that what works for your buddy won't always work for you.

Probably the last (and for some of us, most depressing) lesson from this topic is that if you were born with muscles that are predominantly slow twitch, you are probably never going to be an elite athlete in any sport that requires speed or strength. Yes, you can alter your fiber makeup slightly, but you'll never be as fast or strong as someone who was born that way.

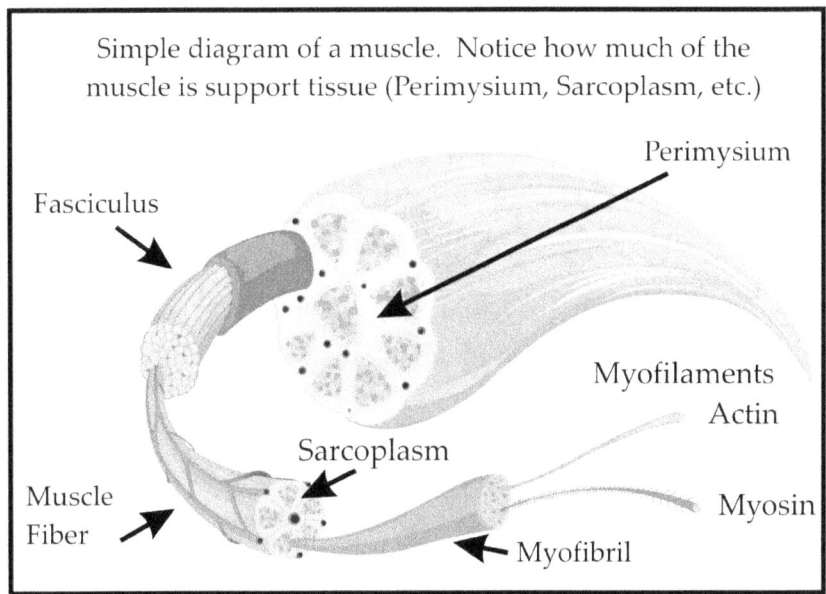

Simple diagram of a muscle. Notice how much of the muscle is support tissue (Perimysium, Sarcoplasm, etc.)

Muscle Growth

There are three ways your muscles can grow: the most common way most adults will put on more muscle is when the individual fibers themselves get bigger. This is called hypertrophy and can further be divided into sarcoplasmic hypertrophy and myofibrillar hypertrophy. The third way is called hyperplasia and is most common through teen years. In the order with which they are most likely to occur, here is an explanation of all three.

Sarcoplasmic Hypertrophy: Produced by high rep training. When muscles grow in this fashion, they are expanding because of an increase in fluid and supportive tissue within the muscle. This is common in endurance athletes, and to an extent, bodybuilders. This type of growth will result in an increase in endurance, as the supportive tissue is better at providing energy to the muscles. This type of growth will show very little increase in strength.

Myofibrillar Hypertrophy: Produced mainly by low rep, high load training. With this type of growth, the muscle cells (fibers) will increase in size. This will result in an increase in strength. This type of growth is common in strength athletes like Olympic lifters, powerlifters, and to some extent bodybuilders (depending on how they train).

Hyperplasia: This type of growth occurs due to an increase in the actual number of muscle cells (fibers). This type of muscle growth is the easiest to maintain, however it occurs mainly in our developmental years, and is rare in adulthood. Some evidence exists that some small amount of hyperplasia will occur in adults that have trained for a long time.

Some conclusions we can draw from this.

- The faster you grow, the less likely you are to be gaining strength and the quicker you will lose this strength.
- If you train as a teen, you will be far more likely to have an increased number of muscle cells, and you will always find it easier to grow and maintain existing muscle (which in part explains my finding that those who are active in youth tend to get back in shape quicker after years of inactivity).
- The longer you train, the easier it will be to stay in shape.
- When you train, even if you are training for size, you still need to decide what type of size you are looking for. Do you want size that will last but take longer to build and will contribute to strength or do you just want the quickest size increase you can get?
- Whether it's because of fiber type or hypertrophy method, you will certainly notice that at a given body fat level, the muscles of a strength athlete will be firmer (even if they are similarly sized) than those of an endurance athlete. This is one of the reasons long, slow cardio is not the way to the

firm "toned" look. In fact, muscle biopsies of endurance athletes will show tissue that looks more like a well-marbled piece of beef while a strength athlete's muscle will look like a lean piece of chicken.

Muscle Shape

You will sometime hear people say: "I want long, lean, firm muscles, not bulky muscles" or "I really want to work on the peak of my biceps." Although you can change the size and firmness of your body parts, the basic shape of your muscles is determined at birth by the length and attachment points of each muscle.

Your muscles attach to your bones through tendons to the origin (side closest to the center of your body) and insertion (end point farthest from the center of your body). These are determined at birth and will not change depending on the exercise you do, nor will the basic shape of your muscles, only the overall size. Sorry, pilates or any other type of exercise will not "give you long, lean muscles." The length and shape of each of your muscles is determined at birth.

Also determined at birth is your potential in any given sport. As with the discussion of fiber type, you may change your overall strength and endurance, but if other athletes have better lever ratios for the needs of a given activity, as determined by limb length and origin and insertion positions, you're probably always going to be second best.

Strength

Your muscle cells are activated by motor neurons. The effectiveness and strength of the firing of these motor neurons IS trainable. An average person may fire their muscles at as little as 50% of their maximum potential simply due to lack of training. An elite athlete may fire their motor neurons at close to 100% effectiveness. This is another reason training age (the number of years you have trained) really matters. As you learn to use your muscles more effectively, you will be able to lift more weight, burn more calories, and grow more muscle.

You've probably noticed that smaller athletes are usually stronger, pound for pound than larger athletes. This isn't some sort of mental Napoleonic complex sort of thing. It's based on solid physics. Strength increases with the square of the size of the muscle because it's dependant on cross sectional area, whereas weight increases with the cube of the size of the muscle because weight is based on volume. Hence weight increases more with size than strength does. To add to that the smaller athlete will have shorter limb lengths and better leverage.

So when someone says something stupid like "an ant is a thousand times stronger than an elephant pound for pound" you'll know why. It's not that the ant's muscle fibers are stronger, just that the elephant is that much bigger and heavier.

The same holds true for strength athletes on a lesser scale, which is why you'll notice that the lighter weight class lifters can lift a great percentage of their body weight. It's not because they are better athletes, just smaller.

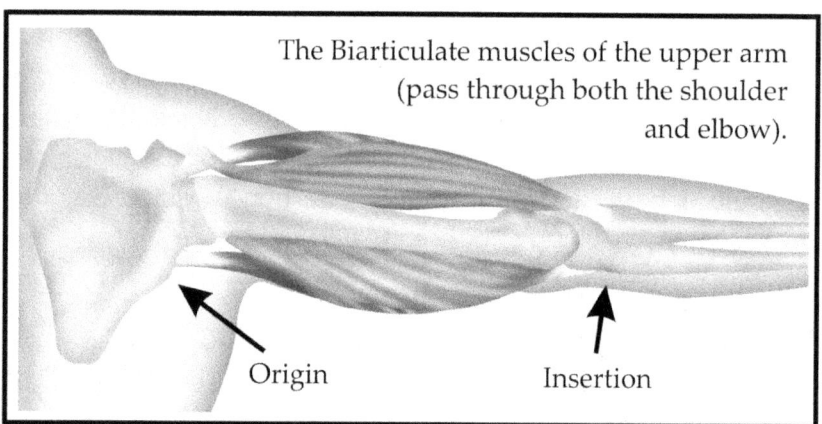

The Biarticulate muscles of the upper arm (pass through both the shoulder and elbow).

Origin   Insertion

Joint Angles

You can probably tell just by looking at your own body that there is not just one muscle controlling the action of each joint in each direction. In fact, in a lot of cases, muscles will pass through two joints (biarticulate) or three joints (triarticulate).

This is useful information because it means that the static angle of one joint may affect the muscle that is used as another adjacent joint is moved. For instance, if you are working your calve muscles with your knees bent, you will primarily be working the soleus muscle because the bent knee loosens the gastrocnemeus so much that it can't be effective, but with a straight leg, the gastrocnemius is the prime mover.

It is also the reason you will see bodybuilders doing curls and tricep exercises from many different positions. The angle of the shoulder changes the overall length of these muscles as they raise and lower the weight.

So you can't just work a particular part of your body with one exercise and position. You have to vary the joint angle of adjacent joints relative to the one worked in order to properly stimulate all of the muscles around that joint.

There you have it: a quick look at how your muscles work. For the physicians out there reading this, I apologize for the over-simplifications and brevity, but hopefully the rest of you have a better idea why your muscles work the way they work. If you'd like to read more, go to www.thinkingpersonsfitness.com for some internet resources that will go deeper into this topic.

Biological Energy Systems

Any system that causes motion requires energy. It would be nice if your body had one simple method for converting the calories you eat into the energy your muscles need, but that's just not the case. Since it isn't so simple, you do need to have some understanding of how your body supplies energy to your muscles in order to maximize the effectiveness of your training. We're going to GREATLY simplify this topic as we did the last, since even a freshman exercise science textbook will spend dozens of pages on this complicated subject.

In simple terms, your body has three ways of providing energy to your muscles, and all three are active during any type of activity, but depending on the duration and intensity of the activity, one of them will predominate. For those who want to look them up, they're called the phosphagen system, glycolysis, and oxidative system. Since glycolysis is functionally a combination of the phosphagen system and the oxidative system, I'm going to simplify them by saying your body provides energy either anaerobically or aerobically.

Aerobic systems require oxygen to function. This is why you breathe harder when you're running. Your body needs oxygen to provide energy to your muscles. Activities lasting longer than 3-5 minutes are almost entirely aerobic.

Short, high intensity activities like a set of chin-ups are anaerobic: your body is not relying on oxygen as part of the process for providing energy. You could do an entire set holding your breath if you wanted to (although not recommended). Any activity lasting less than ten to thirty seconds is almost entirely anaerobic.

Any activity between 30 seconds and 3-5 minutes uses a combination of both the anaerobic and aerobic systems.

This topic is important, because you need to understand what you're trying to train. Remember, your body adapts to the specific stimulus you give it.

Both of your body's energy systems can be trained to be more productive. If you push your body's anaerobic systems, you'll develop the ability to do intense activity harder and for a longer period of time. If you push your aerobic systems, you'll be able to run or bike harder without running out of breath. However, most people who do a lot of cardio don't really push their aerobic capacity. They just go longer at the same intensity. Yes, that may burn calories, but it won't actually increase your aerobic capacity. You won't really be improving anything.

Interval cardio is great for improving aerobic capacity. By varying the length of the intervals, you'll work on improving one or more of your body's energy systems instead of just burning (minimal) calories.

Keep the intervals short and very intense, with plenty of rest between and you'll really push your anaerobic limits. Doing sprints of 50-100 yards where you find yourself slowing down at the end is one good way to push your anaerobic systems. Farmers walks, sandbag carries or pretty much any activity that is short and really intense will work.

Make the intervals longer (2-5 minutes) and you'll work your aerobic systems. Although you won't take yourself completely to the limit like you would in the shorter intervals, you'll still want to push yourself to the point where your heart rate has increased well past the rate it would reach through steady state cardio, and you feel like you can't go farther. You'll want to rest long enough that your heart rate comes back down to the level it would be during steady state cardio, then begin another interval.

There is no way to truly separate your energy systems. Your body will always be utilizing all of its energy systems, and depending on the length of your rest breaks, the shorter intervals will also provide an aerobic workout as well.

The nice thing about these types of energy system workouts is that they will not compromise your physique or overall quality of life goals the way long, steady state cardio will.

Chapter 5 – Resistance Training

Lack of proper resistance training falls only a little behind bad diet as the number one reason why people fail to accomplish their fitness goals.   Without some sort of resistance training, your precious muscle will disappear as you age. The average person will lose about a half pound of muscle per year starting sometime in their mid 20's. Not only will this cause you to slowly loose functionality, but it will also cause you to look "flabby" regardless of your body weight. That half pound per year will also cause the metabolism slowdown so many people consider normal with age.

Also, without stressing your muscles on a regular basis, you will not be stressing your bones either. Without loading your skeletal system, you are increasing your risk of osteopina or osteoporosis as well. The evidence is finally becoming obvious that resistance training is the best method of maintaining strong bones.[13,14,15]

The fact is, if you want to be fit, you MUST incorporate some sort of resistance training into your fitness program.

There are all sorts of ways to do this. Some of them are more convenient or time efficient than others. I encourage you to experiment with many of them. Part of the problem with any exercise program is that for most people, eventually it will get stale and boring.

Also, although a properly designed program will hopefully work all of the muscles from a variety of positions, using completely different methods will always find a way to hit a muscle or two in new and painful ways (good kind of pain of course).

Types of Resistance

Just moving your body using your muscles is not sufficient. You need to provide some type of load that is a significant percentage of your maximum. If you aren't doing something in the area of 80% of your maximum effort, you really aren't loading your muscles, joints and bones enough to do much good.

There are various ways to apply this load and they all have their pluses and minuses.

Free Weights

By far the most convenient and most time efficient way to get your resistance training is with free weights. It's also one of the least expensive. You can get used, adjustable weight dumbbells at a garage sale or used sports equipment store for less than the cost of a couple months of a gym membership. You can store them under a bed or in the corner of a closet.

The list of great bodies that have been built with just such equipment is long indeed. In order to work all the muscles, you'll probably have to combine this setup with body weight exercises, but that's a good thing.

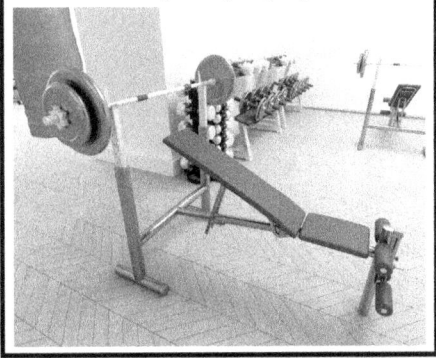

Inexpensive free weights will give you a better workout than much more pricey equipment.

Free weights utilize gravity as the source of resistance. This is good because there is no friction so the eccentric portion of the lift is just as heavy as the concentric portion (very important for both muscle building and fat loss). They also are not stabilized by any means like most machines, so the very important stabilizing muscles will get a workout, and you will not risk pattern overload from repeating a forced motion on your joints.

Free weights have almost no disadvantages other than that you will need to learn how to use them properly to avoid injury.

Well, maybe one other disadvantage. Because there's nothing "new" and "cool" about free weights, you can't impress your friends with the "trendy" new workout program you started.

Body Weight

Exercises such as push-ups, chin-ups, dips, body weight squats (deep knee bends), etc, have been staples of exercise culture for so long for a reason. There is something about using your own body weight for resistance that is just "different."

It's hard to argue with the effectiveness of the basic pushup.

There are quite a few individuals who have built their physiques almost entirely with body weight exercises. Personally, I feel the lack of progressive increase in resistance, and a relatively small amount of possible exercises, makes it advisable to incorporate body weight exercises with free weights, not as a replacement.

Cable Machines

These machines are really just free weights with the resistance redirected with pulleys. They have all the advantages of free weights except for some amount of eccentric robbing friction, which is dependent on the quality of the machine. The better gym quality machines are really good. Some of the home gym type cable setups can have so much friction they become almost unusable.

Since the pulleys redirect the force of gravity, using cable machines enable you to do exercises that are not possible with free weights.

The high cable station on the right, for pull-downs and similar exercises, is a common cable machine that has been around forever.

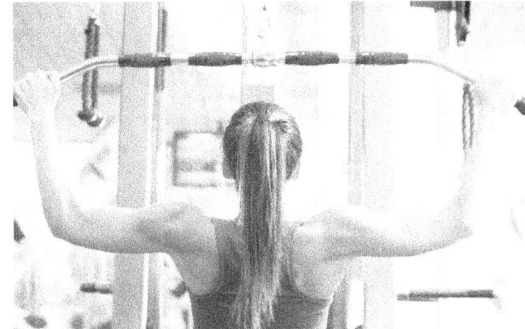

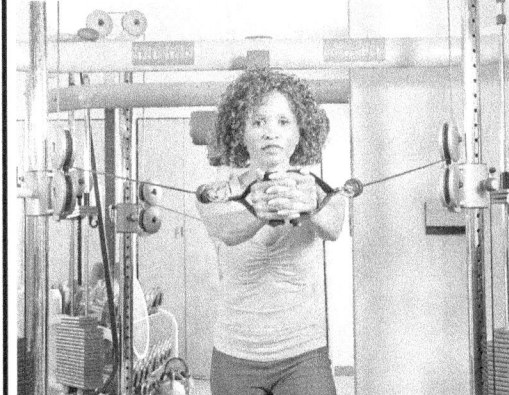

However, there are many types of cable machines such as this highly adjustable dual cable setup, that allows a variety of free weight exercises from many different angles.

Normally, when I'm setting up a "free weight" workout, I will always include some cable based exercises. Most lifters consider cable machines as part of the free weight section of the gym.

Plate Loaded and Weight Stack Machines

These types of machines are like cable machines in that they redirect the force of gravity. Unlike cables, they use various levers to take all the stabilizing effort out of the exercise. They also force the body into a motion that may or may not be natural. Over time, this may cause injury. Friction is also even higher than in most cable machines, resulting in even less eccentric effort (a bad thing for most of us).

If all you're doing is going down the line of machines at the gym, you're not optimizing your progress (if you're making any at all), and wasting a lot of time and effort, as well as setting

If your gym is like most, it's probably full of expensive machines that aren't near as effective as the free weights they tuck away in the back.

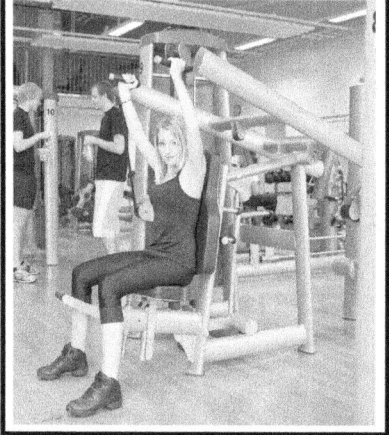

yourself up for injury. I guarantee the guy on the infomercial for those home gym machines did NOT build that awesome body with that machine.

There are some good reasons to use machines to augment your free weight workout. Sometimes certain machines will help you work around an injury, and often, they will allow you to isolate a certain muscle to help you push past a sticking point or force a lagging muscle to grow.

Unlike free weights, cheap machines are usually a recipe for disaster. Do NOT try to setup a home gym with machines!

Exercise Bands

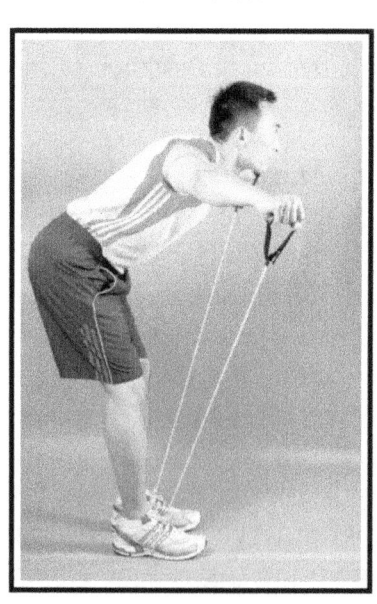

Using elastic tubing for resistance started in physical therapy clinics, probably because it enabled therapists to provide their clients with small amounts of shock free resistance to help rebuild damaged joints and muscles. They work well for this and may be used in a conventional workout program for times and exercises where a cable machine is not practical (traveling for instance).

There are two problems with using exercise bands for

everyday use. First, they provide non-linear resistance. In other words, as you stretch them the resistance increases. You end up with a lot of resistance at the end of the movement and very little at the start. Since muscles will only adapt to a stimulus within 10 degrees of the angle the joint is worked at, this will result in a lack of training effect at the starting end of the movement. Secondly, it is hard to determine how much force is actually being utilized. This makes it very difficult to utilize any sort of progression in your program. This makes progress difficult.

Friction or Hydraulic Machines

These machines are usually found in cheap, women's only gyms, home gyms, and hotel workout rooms. These are at the bottom of the list of methods to get a resistance workout. Other than if you find yourself in a hotel with no other means of working out, you should usually avoid these types of machines. They are difficult to adjust for accurate resistance, making it hard to incorporate progressive resistance increases, and they totally remove the eccentric part of the movement.

The only exception is a few of the high end hydraulic or air based machines that do come in handy for explosive movements without the risk of injury that may come with doing explosive movements with free weights. However you won't see these often, and they're still not the best for general use.

Plyometrics

Plyometrics are usually explosive movements using body weight for resistance. For example, plyometrics would be jumping up onto a box, or jumping back down off the box. For the upper body, clapping push-ups might be a plyometric exercise.

What plyometrics do is enable maximum force to be developed in the muscle in a minimum amount of time. They are very dynamic, and therefore if you are not already reasonably fit, you will risk injuring yourself.

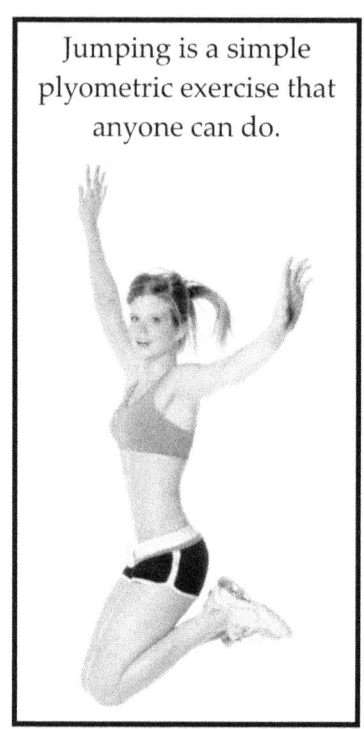

Jumping is a simple plyometric exercise that anyone can do.

Even before the name caught on, plyometrics have long been popular with athletes for good reason: they help develop explosive power, which is not a bad goal for anyone, but certainly not worth risking injury over. For that reason alone, I will not go into plyometrics in this book. By the time you progress to the point where plyometrics will benefit your program (if ever), you will be able to find information on this form of training in a variety of places.

Sports and the Real World

I know some very strong people who have never set foot in a gym. That I can remember, all of them built that strength on a farm or other highly labor intensive job while growing up. Either that or they played very intense sports in their youth. If you've ever spent a day chopping wood, carrying concrete, etc. you know why.

I don't expect anyone to take a job on a farm to get in shape. It's a very inefficient way to get in shape from a time perspective: "sorry boss, I've got to take a break from the Law Firm to get a job that will get me in shape." But you might want to think of this form of exercise the next time you do have a chance to do some heavy real world lifting. Doing it yourself (baring health issues like a bad back or heart) might save you some cash AND time in the gym.

Strongman tools are sometimes a fun way to convert real world work into an interesting workout. They are basically just an artificial way of doing the above: Big truck tire for flipping, rocks for carrying, pushing your car up and down the driveway.

Yes, it sounds weird, but many of us "non-strongmen" find it to be a novel way to get a good workout on a nice sunny day.

Most sports will provide a cardio workout, but some may classify as resistance training. Gymnastics, wrestling and to some extent, dancing and martial arts are some that come to mind. Most aggressive sports provide some sort of lower body resistance training, but only if played aggressively. I think it is a shame that the sports we play become less of a real workout as we get older, but that's the way the world works. Basketball makes way to tennis, then to golf, and soon thereafter, golf with a cart.

I'm not saying everyone reading this needs to go out and take up gymnastics at 45, but it's an important lesson for those with kids. I can always tell to what extent a new client played sports when they were younger. Not just in how fast they get back into shape, but by the "body awareness" they have when their form is critiqued. A guy who played football or wrestled, or a woman who was a competitive gymnast or dancer will almost always succeed in their goals faster than someone who never competed in sports.

Hopefully this section will get you thinking "how can I make my workouts different and fun?" Some people can go through the same old workout day in and day out, and never get bored, and small changes in routine and method allows them to keep advancing.

However, some people can't. They need some variety to keep it interesting. Always keep your eye on fitness magazines or web sites for new and different ways to changeup your workout, but at the same time, keep your eye on the bottom line: how effective are my workouts?

The Stability Continuum – Machines to Swiss Balls

One of the hardest parts about being an instructor of any kind is dealing with fads, gadgets and gimmicks. Regardless of whether you're teaching golf or the piano, every day you'll get a student or prospective student who will approach you asking why you don't incorporate this or that new gadget into their training routine.

What students of each discipline need to understand is that gadgets and gimmicks rarely improve on anything. In the best case, they may help augment existing methods in specific areas, but most of the time, are only invented to make money off gullible people.

Machines

Weight machines have been around for longer than most of us have been alive. Although there may have been others before him, from what I know, the first major introduction of machines into the weight room occurred in 1957 when Harold Zinkin introduced the 'Universal Gym'. I honestly believe his motivation was good. He believed he could make weight lifting safer for people who didn't have the proper training in free weights.

What he didn't realize was that not only were his machines taking most of the smaller, stabilizing muscles out of the action, but they were also possibly causing pattern overload injuries due to the fact that the line of motion was severely, and improperly limited.

Many improvements have been made to weight machines since then, and the newer machines you will see in many gyms are really quite good. Many of them have so many adjustments that they can be made to properly fit people of all shapes and sizes. They also have multiple degree of freedom lever arms that allow the motion to go where you're body wants it to go, not where the machine wants it to go.

Although I don't have any studies to back this up, I would think these newer machines have greatly reduced the incident of pattern overload injuries. I say "greatly reduced" because there are still many motions (like the leg extension) that can result in injuries if done too frequently.

What you have to understand is that ALL machines (other than cable machines), limit the recruitment of the stabilizing muscles to some extent. So yes, while machines may make it easier for beginners to start resistance training without instruction, they will also end up strengthening only the prime movers, and not the stabilizers. This makes it even more likely that these beginners will have injuries in real life or in the gym should they ever try to make the transition to free weights (since the prime movers will be stronger, they will be more likely to attempt weights that the stabilizers will not be able to handle).

Since machines have gotten a bad reputation among the hardcore weightlifters, various manufacturers have attempted to make machines that don't look like machines, usually by eliminating the cable and weight stack and replacing them with somewhere to put standard free weight plates. These are no different from any other weight machine and in many cases worse (since the use of the plates just causes uneven resistance through the range of motion). Probably the most popular of these machines is the Smith machine. This machine allows the lifter to do various barbell based lifts while constraining the weight to a single plain of motion. The lifter gets the ego boost of feeling as if he is using free weights, while getting all the assistance of a standard machine movement.

Regardless of the type of machine, if you rely totally on machines for your resistance training, you are reducing both the effectiveness and overall safety of your workouts.[16],[17]

Notice I excluded cable based machines from my definition of machines? There is a very good reason for this. Cable machines of all types just redirect the force of gravity, allowing movements and muscle angles that would not otherwise be possible. They do not restrict the line of motion or hand position and angle throughout the motion, so they do not suffer from any of the drawbacks of other types of machines. Hence, I do not classify them with other machines. I highly recommend utilizing a good high and low pulley cable machine for many exercises. I said "good" cable machine, because the cheap ones have so much friction that they do not allow any real eccentric resistance.

Sometimes there are good reasons to make use of various machines. There are certainly machines that allow the lifter to work various muscles in a way that is hard to duplicate with free weights (leg curl is a good example). They allow you to move through a workout at a fairly fast pace, and they may allow you to train more effectively around an injury, by isolating out a injured body part that may need some rest.

However, you must be VERY careful not to let the above reasons turn you into a machine junky. Much like anything "easy" in this world, you may quickly find yourself running through the various machines on a daily basis. You will not be doing yourself any favors in the long term.

Of course, you need to stay as far away as possible from the various inexpensive home machines. These are rarely of ANY use and will quickly result in pattern overload injuries. I'll also include the Pilates reformer on this list, as it is a device that has been taken FAR beyond its originally intended use and will result in a blatantly inferior resistance workout.

Unstable Surface Training

In recent years, a new trend has started that goes in the exact opposite direction from machines: unstable training devices. I'm not sure if it is a result of decades of people using machines and the resulting lack of stabilizer training, or just the desire of various uneducated personal trainers trying to compare themselves to physical therapists by attempting (badly) to copy their methods, but unstable training is popping up in the routines of incompetent trainers everywhere.

What I'm talking about is the various balls, boards, and other unstable devices, which the client sits or stands on while doing an exercise. Most of these devices came from physical therapy clinics, where they are more properly used by the therapists for entirely different reasons. They have become very popular recently with trainers, and it seems some excellent and experienced trainers are being viewed as "old school" for not using these devices extensively. Some less than educated trainers do almost their entire sessions with their clients on top of these devices. Trainers will use these devices for a number of reasons.

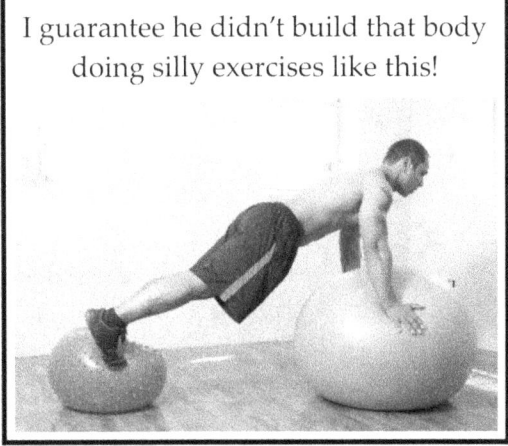

I guarantee he didn't build that body doing silly exercises like this!

For the most part trainers use balance devices because they look cool and they're cheap compared to real exercise equipment, they can carry them from one clients home to another very easily, and many clients find them entertaining. Since the workout is less intense when these devices are used, it appeals to the client's hidden laziness.

Next, when an exercise is performed on a balance device, it then becomes even more complicated and technically difficult. Isn't that a good thing? Well, not really, at least not all the time.

Actually, the more unstable the body is during an exercise, the more the brain shuts down the muscles that are most responsible for the movement. So, let's say you do a standard squat. In that exercise, the quads, glutes, etc, get a major workout. Now, do the same exercise on top of a bosu ball, and these big muscles only fire at half their potential, and therefore don't get near the workout.

Instead, smaller stabilizing muscles will get a much greater workout, and that's not necessarily a bad thing, but if the majority of your workout is done this way, you will not get nearly as good of a workout for the big muscles (the ones you actually see, and do most of the work, and burn most of the calories).

So you might say "I'll just use machines for my big prime mover muscles, and then unstable training devices to hit the stabilizing muscles." Well, that MIGHT work, or you could just use free weights in the first place and work them all at once.

Another reason balance training is often used by the uneducated trainer is to improve sports performance. Unfortunately, in the majority of cases, this is also refuted by exercise science. Studies have repeatedly demonstrated that the body does not improve its ability to balance on a steady surface by practicing on an unstable surface (think about how off balance you are on land after a couple days on a cruise ship). In fact, a few studies have suggested that training on an unstable surface may actually decrease performance on a stable surface, and let's face it, the vast majority of sports are performed on solid ground.

This actually makes sense when you think about all that goes into balance. Your eyes, inner ears, and muscle proprieceptors all coordinate to allow your brain to balance properly. Throw one of these signals out of whack (which is what you're doing on an unstable surface) and your body will decondition its normal balance mechanism. So, practicing your golf swing on top of an unstable surface will probably not help your swing unless you're going to go golfing on the deck of a cruise ship out at sea (unstable surface).

However, if you're developing your balance skills for snowboarding (unstable environment) then a balance board of some sort may be perfect training. As usual, you need to evaluate why something is done, not just whether it looks neat or whether everyone else is doing it!!!

So there you have it. At one end are machines, which are overly stabile and restrictive, and on the other end unstable training devices which will give the stabilizing muscles a real workout, but won't give you near as good of an overall workout. There are uses for the entire spectrum but just make sure you understand why you are using a certain device and as with most of life, moderation is key. Stick with the middle ground (free weights) for most of your program.

A "Bongo Board" is great training if you're into skateboarding, surfing, or snowboarding.

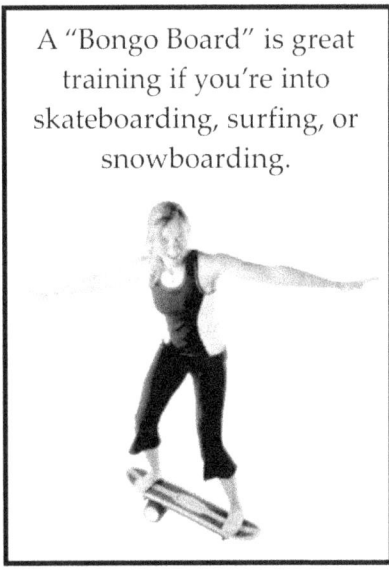

Chapter 6 - Workout Programming

"Everything should be made as simple as possible, but not simpler." — *Albert Einstein*

KISS (Keep It Simple Stupid). It's an adage you should keep in mind when working out. Yes, you could find a new workout program for every day of the week. Most of them are written by gurus who swear this workout is the best and perhaps only way to achieve your goals.

While it's nice that people are thinking of new ways to keep working out fresh and interesting, the fact is, there are relatively few principles that really matter, or at least that matter to someone who isn't dedicating their life to their physique.

In any subject, there are always little details that will perhaps gain someone a one-half of one percent advantage. In stock car racing, an increase of one horsepower is a big deal. That's only about 1/600th of the total power output, but to them, it makes a difference. However you'd never notice that difference in your daily driver or even your weekend hotrod.

Unfortunately, those tiny, useless details are the ones that sell magazines. Hence, they seem to be the factors most people spend all their time on.

As I write this, one of the most popular workouts going around is so complicated and so "all over the place," that it easily spends 50% of the workout time on insignificant but time consuming exercises. Yes, if you follow this program, you will see results, but you'll spend 30-50% more time doing it than you would if you just stuck with the simple, but effective, basics.

At the end of the chapter, I will provide some instruction on the primary exercises, but in order to keep this book from being a 500 page encyclopedia of exercises, you will need to refer to other sources for most of the listed exercises. I will try to keep the names consistent to the names used elsewhere, but many exercises have multiple names. Several good (and free) sources are listed on my web site.

Now that I just got done telling you to keep it simple, I'm going to talk a little about workout construction. I'm going to try to keep each part as uncomplicated as possible, and just give you the info you'll need to construct a basic workout program on your own (or determine the quality of a workout you see elsewhere).

Exercise Selection: Big vs. Small Exercises

Probably the most obvious mistake I see in gyms everywhere is simply bad choices of exercises. The guy who's 100 lb's overweight and spends 15 minutes doing bicep curls is pretty obvious, but did you realize that the same individual spending 15 minutes doing crunches is making an equally bad choice?

I see it all the time: someone in the gym who is out of shape and doing a bunch of small isolation exercises (ex. bicep curls, tricep kickbacks). Yes, they're a lot easier, and don't take near as much out of you, but that's the point and the problem. You NEED to be doing the exercises that really "take it out of you."

These "bigger" exercises also work many more muscles at once. A couple sets of free weight squats will do the work of a half dozen machine based leg exercises. Squats, deadlifts, lunges, presses, rows and similar exercises should make up the core of your program. Save the isolation exercises for the competitive bodybuilder, or other advanced lifter who has distinct areas they need to work on.

You've heard it before, but most of you still refuse to believe it. There's no such thing as spot reduction! There's nothing wrong with including some crunches in your program, but don't think they're going to help with that beer gut. Stick with the big exercises that build muscle and burn calories. We've all got a six pack. For most people it's just buried under a layer of fat.

You may also want better, firmer arms, but a bunch of curls aren't going to help them until you get your body fat to a reasonable level.

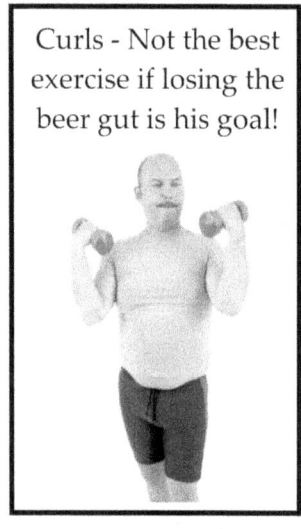

Curls - Not the best exercise if losing the beer gut is his goal!

Another less obvious error I see in exercise selection is lack of balance. I go into this more under the posture section, but I can't count the number of hard working, otherwise experienced exercisers who are obviously ignoring several very important muscle groups. Follow my recommendations in the "Your First Workout" section, and balance in exercise selection won't be a problem.

If you have a couple years under your belt, you may start to notice you are strong in some areas and weak in others. Remember, everybody is different. There is no way I can set out an exercise routine that is going to be completely balanced for everyone.

For instance, many people will never have to do isolation work for their arms. Yes, that's right, for many goals curls and tricep extensions may be a total waste of your time. However, once you progress, you may notice that your arms do need a little extra work, either because other lifts such as pull-ups or bench presses are being held back by a lack of arm strength, or because aesthetically you feel your physique could use more.

At the point where you are aware of your strengths and weaknesses, you'll be able to add a set here or there or subtract a set from some muscle groups. Just make sure you are being honest: don't stop doing squats because you think your quads are too big when the real reason is that you hate squats!!!

Choose you exercises for specific reasons, not because you like them or don't like them. Make sure you're always balancing your program and are not just concentrating on the muscles you can see in the mirror.

Progression

If you're doing the same routine you were doing a year ago, don't be surprised if you're in the same shape you were in a year ago.

Whether it's increasing the weight you use, the number of reps, or the number of sets, if you're workouts are not getting tougher, then neither are you. Your body will adapt only to new stimuli.

Sometimes the new stimulus can be a completely new workout program, but from week to week you'll need to make smaller changes as well. Planning for small increments in weight on each exercise is probably the best way to do this, but in the beginning, you'll also find yourself able to add more sets to each workout.

Of course, in order to keep your workouts time efficient, you won't want to add sets indefinitely. At some point you'll have to rely on weight and intensity increases.

Unfortunately, as far as progression is concerned, people either don't use the concept or they over use it. As with a lot of life, moderation is the key here.

Not to over generalize, but it seems people who have been told they need to add resistance training to their cardio workouts, tend to ignore the need for progression. They'll do the same workout day in and day out, never adding weight or intensity. After a couple months, they quit resistance training completely because they can't figure out why it didn't do anything for them.

Then there's the guy who jumps into resistance training really desiring strength and muscle increases. He watches the guy next to him benching three times as much as he can, so he adds a 25lb plate to the bar on every workout. Then he's surprised when he blows out his shoulder a month into his program.

Remember, you're in this for life. You'll be amazed how quickly the first year passes, and how much total progress you'll make. Just keep the progression small and steady.

Full Body vs. Split Routines

A split routine is one in which only part of the body is worked in any given workout. The theory is that it enables you to concentrate more on that particular body part. The most common type of split is an upper/lower body split. For example, you might work the upper body on Monday and Thursday, and the lower body on Tuesday and Friday.

The vast majority of serious athletes and bodybuilders use split routines most of the time. However, I don't advocate a split routine for most of the people reading this book. I feel a split routine has more disadvantages than advantages for the average person who is just looking to get in shape:

1. You need to be hitting the weights at least four times a week with a split routine. If you're only doing two or three weight workouts a week, half or all of your body is only getting worked once a week. This allows too much recovery time, and you end up backsliding.

2. For weight loss or beginning muscle building, you really need to be stimulating the muscle every 48 hours or so. More recovery than that, and your body stops compensating (recovering from the last workout) and your metabolism slows down. For strength gains, weightlifters may need longer between workouts for optimum neurological recovery, but most of us aren't competitive weightlifters.

3. In the beginning, you'll have enough trouble with muscle soreness, even with full body routines. If you start out with a split routine, you may soon find that walking or combing your hair becomes next to impossible the day after a workout. A competitive bodybuilder might come away from a "leg day"

106

hardly able to walk. Most of us have real lives! Some of us would actually like to be able to function the next day! For beginning muscle growth and weight loss, as well as general fitness, we don't need to do such devastating workouts.

On many occasions I'll recommend a program that will have an "exercise split". By using alternate exercises every other workout we are hitting the entire body each workout, but in a different way. I feel this is the best of both worlds for most people.

Don't take this to mean that split workouts aren't of any use. At a certain level they're almost required, but certainly not for everyone. At what level do you move to split workouts? I would say the primary indication that you need to make the switch is when you feel you are no longer making progress with three or four full body resistance training sessions per week.

I strongly believe that for general fitness, health, and quality of life as we age, three GOOD full body sessions per week should be enough. If you decide you want to be a little more "muscular" than just "fit", you may certainly need to step up to more frequent split workouts.

Sets and Reps

This is one of the subjects that everyone makes such a huge deal about. Yes, it does matter, but it's really not as complicated or technical as they make it sound.

First, number of sets: Someone released one of those studies I complained about in the beginning of the book stating all anyone ever needs is one set. I won't go into the reasons the study was flawed, but to make a long subject short, several studies have been done since showing more sets are usually better.

The most typical set rep scheme is 3x10, or 3 sets of 10 reps. The gurus' always make fun of this set/rep scheme, but there's a reason it's been around forever: it works. Three sets just seems to be the right amount for many different goals. Not all goals, mind you, and not all the time, but as a general rule, I find it takes at least one set to get up to speed with the exercise. Whether it's priming the nervous system or getting the muscles loose and "into the grove" it really doesn't matter. You're first set will never be the best. The second set should be a very good work set, and the third set should exhaust the muscle to some reasonable extent.

For some assistance exercises (curls, shrugs, calve raises), I may only do one or two sets, and if I'm training for strength, I may do 5 or more sets, with none of them to failure. Generally speaking, the higher your reps, the lower the number of sets, although this too is not always true.

The number of reps you do in each set can be constant, or can change. Some people like to make a big deal out of this, but I don't feel it really matters, as long as you're ramping up to the final set. I often use less weight on the first set, and just do whatever number of reps allows me to feel ready for the main sets, but it really depends on the exercise. If you're doing squats, then starting low is generally good. If it's your 3rd upper or lower body exercise of the day, then a warm-up is probably unnecessary.

There are more set/rep schemes than I can mention: 5x5 for strength, ramping the weight up or down, usually ramping the reps in the opposite direction; pyramiding, where you ramp up then back down (either weight or reps), etc.

Many people really obsess over this, but I think the most important point with sets and reps is not that there is any magic number for either sets or reps, but that you change things up every once in a while. Find something that works for you, but don't be afraid to try something different.

Arranging Your Sets

How you arrange your sets can be important to the specific goals you have set for yourself.

Straight Sets

Straight sets are as simple as they sound. If you're doing three sets of each exercise, you simply do three sets of one exercise, then move to another exercise. Straight sets are used most often when strength or muscle gains are the main priority. They have the huge disadvantage of being very time consuming, since you must rest between each set. Workouts will take up to twice as long when you utilize straight sets, and you will get very little energy system work with straight sets.

I almost never utilize straight sets for an entire workout. About the only time I use them is for big exercises at the beginning of a split workout. For instance, if I'm doing "Leg Day" I might start the workout with five straight sets of squats before moving into the rest of my workout arranged in Supersets.

Superset

A superset is one in which you alternate between two or more exercises. I like alternating between unrelated muscle groups to give each muscle time to recover from each set. This way I can move quickly between each set.

I'm a huge proponent of supersetting your workouts. Not only does it allow you to do more work in less time, but it also gives you an energy system workout at the same time. Usually not much of an aerobic system workout, but definitely an anerobic energy system workout. For a competitive weightlifter or most bodybuilders, this would be counterproductive. They want to make sure their body and mind are almost completely rested between sets. Their workouts will often last more than an hour, and many will do two workouts per day.

But you're not a competitive weightlifter or bodybuilder. If you were, you wouldn't be reading this book. You're a busy person with a life, a job, kids, etc. The object here is to get you as fit as possible in as little time as possible.

Circuits

Circuits are simply an extension of Supersets. Instead of alternating between two or three exercises, you'll go through your complete workout one exercise at a time, one set of each. Once you are done with the circuit, you'll start over and do it again. There is really no defined advantage to circuits, other than to just mix things up a bit and, if done fast enough, really hit your energy systems hard.

Complexes

Complexes have been around for a while, but are seeing a huge increase in popularity lately. A complex is very much like a circuit, with a series of perhaps a half dozen exercises done in series without rest, except that they are all done with the same barbell or dumbbells without ever setting them down.

A sample complex might be:

Stiff leg deadlifts

Front squats

Bent over rows

Push presses

Shoulder shrugs

These complexes are extremely energy system intensive, and when done properly will really help strip off the body fat, but they have several very distinct disadvantages:

Complexes must be constructed and performed properly. Very few people seem to have the expertise to set up complexes correctly. The results of an improperly designed complex workout are the same as an improperly designed workout of any other type: injury, muscle imbalances, lack of progress, etc.

If complexes are badly setup or performed improperly, bad form can creep in very quickly, even on exercises where you are otherwise very familiar. Since the fatigue is so extreme, it is very easy to let your form slip. Injury will result much sooner than with other methods.

For this reason, I recommend complexes only for advanced trainers who are already in very good condition, have a mastery of exercise form, and no nagging injuries. Even so, for most, complexes offer no real advantages over combining conventional lifting with interval cardio, but if you're looking for an interesting change to your established routine, they may be useful.

Dumbbells vs. Barbells

I am personally a big fan of dumbbells, especially for upper body movements. If you are a powerlifter or an ordinary gym rat whose ego is based on his max bench press, you can probably ignore this topic, but if you are the average client I train and are more concerned with how you look and feel than what kind of numbers you lift, I feel you'll be much better served by dumbbells.

The reason is simple. With a barbell, your hands are tied together and constrained in how they can move throughout the lift. Similar to machines, this will force your shoulders and elbows to move through a pattern that is not truly natural (your hands are not allowed to rotate in any direction, forcing your elbows and shoulders to compensate). Over years of lifting, it is quite probable you will suffer pain and/or injuries to these joints. I know very few hardcore benchers that don't develop rotator cuff injuries, and only then make the switch to dumbbells. Most of them will then tell you they wish they had made the switch years ago.

Notice how the angle of the hands are constrained in the barbell bench press on the left, whereas they are free to rotate to a more natural position in the dumbbell bench press on the right.

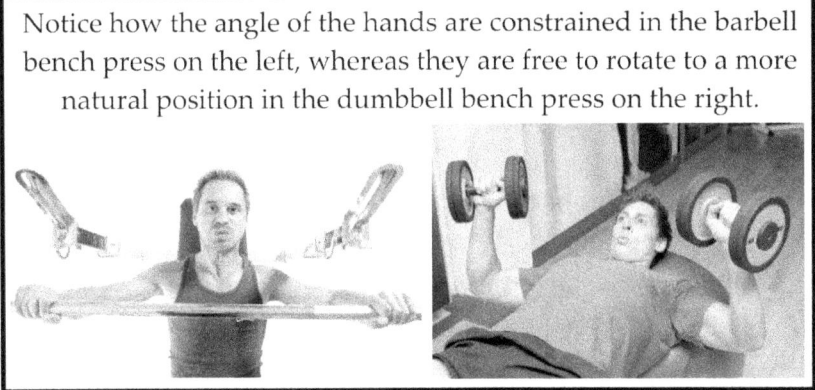

By using dumbbells, the hands are allowed to move separately, and if done properly, the shoulders and elbows will not develop pattern overload injuries. Dumbbells will also activate the stabilizing muscles better, since it is more difficult to control two separate weights than one big weight that is tied together in the center.

I am not by any means warning against the use of barbells. I understand that pressing with dumbbells may not result in the same amount of activation of some muscles as will the same exercise with a barbell, and for many that is a big factor. Also, some people MAY have adequate range of motion such that problems will not occur.

Dumbbells will also force you to even out any strength discrepancies from arm to arm. With a barbell, slight changes in the way you lift can move a lot of the weight from your weak side to your strong side, perpetuating imbalances.

It's been years since I picked up a barbell for upper body work, and although I can no longer tell you how much I bench (like that ever really mattered), my workouts and physique have not suffered in the least, and my shoulders are much happier.

Unilateral vs. Bilateral

A unilateral exercise is one that works only one arm or leg at a time. Bilateral works both at once.

Bilateral exercises are the traditional squats, deadlifts, stiff leg deadlifts, etc. The big advantage of these are that you can simply lift more weight that way as there is less balance and stabilization necessary. Some trainers will even go so far as to say that lower body bilateral training is unessesary. I disagree. Everytime I've taken a break from bilateral work for any significant amount of time, I've always regreted it as my overall strength has declined.

Unilateral vs. bilateral, particularly for the lower body, is a similar issue to dumbbells vs. barbells, as the unilateral exercises (single leg squats, lunges, sprinter squats, single leg SL deadlift)

Single Leg (unilateral) Deadlift, Squat and Elevated Split Squat

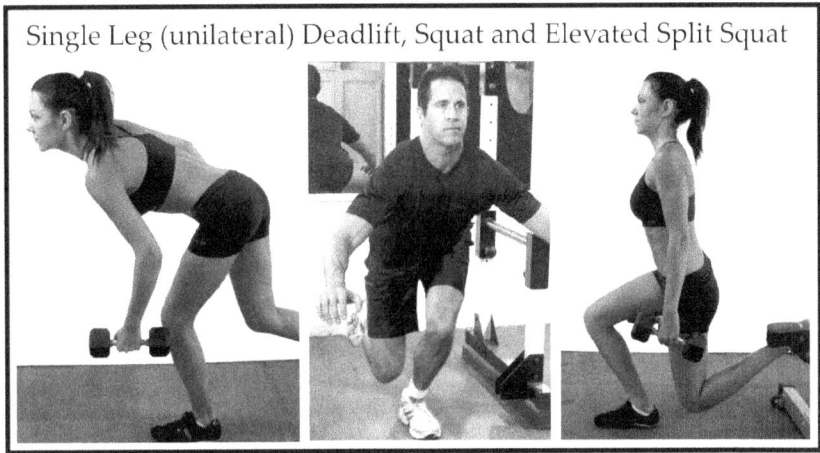

are tremendously useful in working the stabilizers, especially at the knee, but do not allow near the weight to be used, resulting in much less recruitment of the prime movers.

I like to incorporate some amount of unilateral work in my programs during all phases. Sometimes after the big lifts (squats or deads), and sometimes on a one-on, two-off program where you'll do unilateral exclusively in one out of every three of your leg workouts.

I also find them very useful in cutting phases (dropping fat) where I'm trying to move through many exercises quickly. I'll combine unilateral movements (which require little setup since they use dumbbells) with machines like leg press and leg curl. This gives my body a rest from squatting and deadlifting for a while, yet still hits both the prime movers and stabilizers.

It is also helpful to use some unilateral exercises in your upper body routine as well. Virtually any upper body exercise can be done unilaterally by just picking up one dumbbell instead of two, or using a single-handed pulley handle. Although doing so will not change the exercise as fundamentally as it will with lower body exercises, you will notice a difference in how the muscles are getting worked, and often, you'll find you get a rather interesting core workout from the effect of maintaining side to side stability with a weight in only one hand.

Intensity of sets and reps

I've already talked about the necessity for intensity in your workouts, but how do you get that intensity, and how much at what times? Of course intensity is relative for each individual. I can tell one person to "take the set to failure" and get a totally different level of exertion than if I said the same to another person.

Although many people are chronically deficient in workout intensity, it's impossible to use 100% intensity all of the time. Knowing when to go all out and how to do it safely is very important.

There are three types of intensity: Intensity of the rep, set and workout. You may have different levels of intensity within each workout. An Olympic weightlifter may use maximum intensity on each rep, but stop each set and each workout well short of failure. This athlete needs to be able to train as much and as often as possible. He uses maximum intensity for each rep because there is no other way he will improve, but if he took each set or workout to failure, he wouldn't be able to train nearly as often.

Intensity in each rep can of course be increased by increasing the weight, but it can also be increased by concentrating on accelerating the weight as fast as possible. Push as hard as possible, even if the weight itself is less than the maximum weight you can lift.

If you are not training for strength exclusively or have not been training for very long, I advise keeping the intensity of each rep rather low. The intensity of a set will vary depending on the goals of that set, and how much fatigue you can tolerate.

Pre-Failure

The vast majority of your sets will not be to failure or beyond. Despite what some might tell you, it's simply not possible or reasonable to expect your body to constantly perform at that level. That's not to say you'll be wimping out on most of your sets, but they won't be done at maximum intensity. Warm-up sets should obviously not be done to failure.

If you are training for strength, it's usually advisable to rarely take the set to failure. Most strength coaches will advise you to stop each set when the speed of movement starts to slow. So for instance, you might do a set of four with a weight that you could actually do five or six reps, but by stopping at 4 reps, you'd be able to do quite a few sets without tiring. Each rep would be with maximum force (maximum intensity), but at no time during any particular set would you not be able to do another rep.

Failure

Some of your workout sets will certainly be to failure. Again, failure has different definitions to different people, but most commonly it means that you could not have done another rep with good form. Notice I said "good form."

There are some exercises where it is just not possible to go to failure without a spotter. With squats, or bench presses, going to failure without someone to help you out would have bad consequences possibly including injury and embarrassment.

The more experienced you are in the gym, the closer you will be able to get to failure without actually missing a rep. For the most part, if you can get within a rep of true failure, you're probably accomplishing about the same thing. If your goals require more intensity, you're probably going to want to go beyond failure anyway.

Beyond Failure

How can you possibly go beyond failure? It does sound like those coaches on TV that talk about giving 110%. Like wouldn't that make 110% the new 100%? What we're really talking about is using a couple of techniques to extend a set beyond what you could do normally. The reason we would do this is in an attempt to completely exhaust every muscle fiber used in the exercise.

Obviously, the harder you push your muscles, the more they will adapt. It would seem like your body would call every muscle fiber into action at the end of a set, when you can no longer do another rep, but that's seldom the case.

For anyone but an elite trained athlete, your body is usually always holding something back. There are many reasons for this including your nervous system being untrained and inefficient, but the end result is that the only way to truly tax your muscles to their limit is to take a set beyond failure. Here are some methods:

Spotter: Obviously, if you have a workout partner, they can help you get a few more reps by providing a little help on the last couple reps. This is certainly the easiest method, but suffers from several disadvantages including conflicting goals, fitness levels, and having to deal with TWO people's time constraints. In many hard-core weightlifting gyms, asking for a spot from a complete stranger is very normal. I've found most people in your average gym don't want to be bothered.

Drop sets: The next easiest way to go beyond failure is to decrease the weight slightly after you cannot do another rep. Of course this requires you to stop the set, change plates or dumbbells and restart the set. If you move fast enough, it can work reasonably effectively on some exercises, especially any exercise where you are standing and using dumbbells, like curls, military presses, lunges, etc. "Running the rack" is a term used to describe the often-used practice of drop setting curls with dumbbells (40's, 35's, 30's, 25's, 20's, 15's then find someone to help you comb your hair the next day because you can't lift your arms above your shoulders!).

Complexes or switching exercises: Another technique is to setup a complex or circuit of exercises that all use the same main muscle, but in order of decreasing effort. An example for triceps might be skull crushers, followed by close grip bench press, then put down the bar and do a set of push-ups, then end with push-ups from your knees.

Cheat Sets: Many people do this without even realizing that's what they are doing. They let their form deteriorate at the end of a set in order to squeeze out one more rep. Although some advanced lifters, including Arnold, are proponents of this technique, I recommend against it in most exercises. The chance for injury is simply too high. There are better methods of achieving your goals.

ALL of these techniques should be used sparingly. Going beyond failure is very tiring on the neurological system, and doing this too often will keep you from maximizing the effectiveness of the rest of your workout. I can't give you any hard data on how much or how often as it is different for everyone. It will depend on how long you've been training and how fast your body recovers. Doing one set beyond failure for each muscle group is probably appropriate for most people. If you find that you're not recovering as well from your workouts once you start utilizing these techniques, then you're probably overdoing it.

Finally, there's overall workout intensity. How completely exhausted are you after a workout? How badly do your muscles hurt the day after? More is not always better. I feel completely devastating workouts have their place with advanced lifters or those with fast recovery, however for many people, especially those of us who aren't 20 anymore and aren't on performance enhancing drugs, pushing a workout to the point where you can't walk or need to throw up, just isn't productive.

Not only will you need far too much time to recover from a workout of this type, you're quality of life outside the gym will suffer, injuries are much more likely, and the quality of each set will deteriorate as you near the end of the workout.

Intensity of a given workout can be increased by either shortening the rest breaks or increasing the number of sets or the intensity of each set.

Regardless of how you achieve an adequate intensity level of your sets reps or entire workouts, this is a topic that is VERY important. Most people new to working out and who don't have a background in athletics are not using even close to enough intensity. I've watched some newbies waste an hour or more on a workout that lacked sufficient intensity to make any progress at all. However some, particularly young men, will often overdo it. Finding the "sweet spot" for you is important.

Time Between Sets

You will always be taking some sort of rest break between sets. It may just be long enough to move to the next exercise, but it is the break that your body needs to replenish your anaerobic and neurological systems. Without that break, your workouts would be far less effective.

But how long should you take between sets to optimize your progress? It really depends on the goal of the workout.

Competitive weightlifters, who are concerned mainly with training for maximum strength, and therefore place a lot of value on complete neurological recovery between sets, will often take 5 minutes or more between sets.

A bodybuilder who wants to maximize muscle growth, and doesn't care how long he has to spend in the gym, would normally take anywhere from 3-4 minutes between sets.

You've noticed I'm a big fan of supersetting, which allows an individual muscle a couple of minutes between sets, but gives your entire system as little as a minute or less between sets. This is probably not optimum for muscle growth, but from my experience, the tradeoff is worth it.

By supersetting your exercises, you greatly shorten the time you spend in the gym, give your anaerobic energy system a good workout, and even get a moderate aerobic workout. Most of you are not looking for the pro bodybuilder look anyway. If time and efficiency is important to you, keeping the time between exercises short and using supersets to give each muscle a break is probably your best choice.

However, if you do have the time on a particular day, and there's an exercise you really want to maximize, it's not a bad idea to do 5-6 straight sets with 3-4 minutes between sets. I do this a lot with squats and deadlifts.

Concentric vs. Eccentric and Lifting Speed

The speed at which you lift the weight is another subject given way more thought than it needs. There are more theories than there are facts to support the theories, but here are some quick thoughts.

Concentric lifting speed is the speed at which you lift the weight. Eccentric is the speed at which you lower it. In a machine or pulley exercise, the direction may be reversed, but the definition holds true as long as you think of it as you moving the weight during the concentric part of the lift and the weight moving you during the eccentric part.

I will start by saying you should always use a speed that allows you to properly control the weight. Lowering the weight too fast is an easy way to injure yourself.

The faster you lift the weight, the more force you will have to use. Weightlifters who are looking for maximum strength gains will try to lift the weight as quickly as possible for this reason. Slower concentric speeds are usually better for muscle growth.

The eccentric part of the lift should be a little slower and controlled. Many people will sometimes incorporate very slow eccentrics into their program on occasion, as it may result in better muscle growth and more calories burned to recover from the workout as a slow eccentric has been shown to cause increased muscle microtrauma.

This makes slow, controlled eccentrics very important if fat loss is important to you. It's theorized that most of the muscle microtrauma that causes your body to burn so many calories recovering from a workout are as a result of the eccentric part of the lift. This is one of MANY reasons those "women's only" facilities with their hydraulic based equipment are such a bad option: There's no eccentric part at all, and weight loss is by far the number one reason women join these places.

Overall, my advice is to just make sure you're lifting the weight in a controlled mannor, and lower it in a controlled mannor, at least a little slower than you lifted, and perhaps much slower on occasion for an extra "burn".

I do not recommend that you try to count seconds as you raise and lower the weight as recommended by others. This is the last thing you should be concentrating on.

Periodization

Periodization is the process of varying training protocols or training intensity at regular intervals to bring about optimal gains.

The logic behind this is two-fold. First, the body can only adapt to a limited number of goals at once, and second, at some point your body will adapt to a specific training routine, and stop adapting. Some will also preach that periodization is necessary to give the body a break from hard training, by planning regular rest weeks or bouts of lower intensity training, but unless you are a pro athlete training eight hours a day, six days a week, this is usually unnecessary.

How important periodization is to your program will depend a lot on how long you've been training or how advanced you are. If you are out of shape, or just starting out with this program, you will probably not need to worry about it for many months. Your body will be so confused by the very fact that you're working out at all, that gains will continue to come for some time.

In the beginning, you'll be able to lose fat, gain muscle, get stronger and gain endurance, all at the same time. Once you have some time in, it becomes very hard to lose weight at the same time as you put on muscle, or as you really get advanced, it'll become next to impossible to make improvements in more than one or two body parts at a time! You will need to adjust your program just to maintain your current status, and put emphasis on one part that is lagging, or to improve one specific strength or endurance goal.

This type of periodization is necessary at some point. Don't worry about it if you are just starting out. With time, you'll realize when this approach is necessary.

When some form of periodization is necessary, it can be as simple as just changing your routine every couple of months, or as complicated as rotating through intensity and goals every week on a predetermined program.

On the simple side, there tends to be two types of gym goers: Those who do the same workout day in, day out, year after year, and those who change their workout every time they pick up a new fitness magazine and see a new workout article.

Changing things up is important. If you keep doing the same routine, your body will adapt to it, and the gains will slow or stop completely. How often you change plans is up to you, but I'd always recommend giving any new plan at least a month. After that, you'll know when it's time to change to a new workout, because the progress will stop, or you'll be so bored of the old workout, that you just can't keep the intensity up.

If a plan is working for you, you can often keep it going for many months just by changing small details of the plan as discussed previously or as demonstrated in the workouts chapter.

From there, periodization can get really complicated if you let it (not usually necessary unless you're a pro athlete). Rotating goals or intensity levels from week to week may be something you enjoy doing if you just like to make things complicated, but for the vast majority of trainees, it is unnecessary.

About the only time I find this necessary for non-pro athletes, is when pushing maximum strength. If you are bound and determined to push your bench press or squat higher, then rotating intensity levels from week to week, or workout to workout can give your joints and connective tissue time to adapt and recover, as they will usually adapt much slower than your muscles will.

However, this is of little use if you are sticking to more than 5-6 reps in each set (probably a good thing for the goals of most that are reading this).

Others will also advocate a regular back off, or active rest week. I've found that for most people, planning a rest week during a time when they could be working out on a regular basis, just ends up being frustrating.

This is not to say that a rest week every once in a while is a bad idea. However, what I've found with the busy people I train is that this will happen without any planning at all. There will be an occasional week where working out is just not convenient, and that's a great time to take a break. Maybe while you're on a cruise or touring Paris, or just while you have a cold or injury.

Forcing a rest week, when you could be working out, is usually not necessary. However, if you find you are burned out, tired all the time, not making any progress, have sore joints, or just dreading each trip to the gym AND you've gone several months without missing more than a couple of workouts, then sure, take a week off and see what happens.

Pretty much all of the studies on periodization have been done on professional athletes for good reason: they are the ones who really need it. They're working out or training perhaps upwards of 8-10 hours per day and have very complicated goals. They are so advanced that making even a 1% gain is huge, and it is almost impossible for them to improve on more than one aspect of their conditioning at one time. Their lives revolve around training and competition and back off or rest periods, particularly before competitions, are an absolute necessity, but as with all of this, don't let someone try to persuade you that something that works for a pro athlete is going to necessarily work for you.

So now you have the basic knowledge to construct your own workout programs or at least pick a quality workout from a bad one. I've tried to keep it as simple as possible, but at the same time, I feel I've given you as much detail as you'll need. Unless you decide to change careers and become a fitness model, you'll probably never need to get any more sophisticated than this.

Chapter 7 – Cardio

Ok, I'll admit that I HATE CARDIO! Unless it's in the form of a sport or activity like Mountain Biking, Rollerblading, or Basketball, there's very little I like less than to spend my time sitting on an exercycle or plodding along on a treadmill. Even with a TV or book in front of me, I still find it to be a monotonous activity.

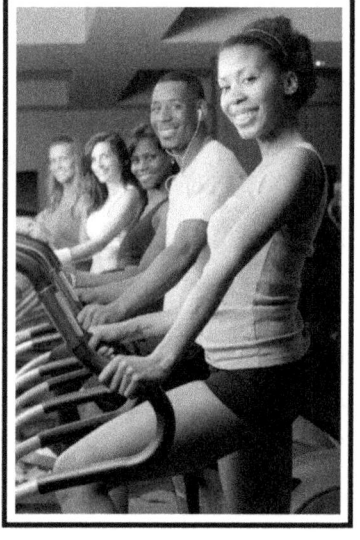

Why don't the people I see plodding along on the treadmills look this fit OR this happy?

Having said that, unless you're a powerlifter who doesn't care about your health or ability to walk up a set of stairs without needing to catch your breath at the top, cardio is important, and needs to be part of your workout routine.

Ironically, there doesn't seem to be much in the way of "in between" as far as cardio is concerned. There are people like me, who have to drag themselves onto the stairstepper when the roads are covered with ice, or those who just seem to love to log hour after hour on a treadmill.

Twenty years ago, it would have been blasphemy to suggest someone was doing too much cardio, but for many goals, it is often the case. This is a topic that will get some people's "undies in a bunch" but at the risk or upsetting some of you, I will say that many die-hard exercise nuts really overdo the cardio. As amazing as it sounds, even Dr. Kenneth Cooper, the father of the aerobic fitness revolution is now advocating people be careful how much cardio they do and make sure to get enough resistance training.[18]

Too Much Cardio?

What is "too much cardio?" I would define it as doing more cardio than is productive for your stated goals.

First, some definitions: Many people (including me at this point) use the terms "cardiovascular exercise", and "aerobic exercise" interchangeably. Although they do overlap to some extent, they are not precisely the same thing. In very simple terms, cardiovascular exercise is exercise that improves the performance (health) of the heart and circulatory system. Aerobic exercise is exercise that improves ones aerobic capacity, or the ability of your body to process oxygen and deliver it to the muscles doing the work.

In a sense, aerobic is a broader term than cardiovascular. aerobic exercise encompasses cardio exercise. The heart is a big part of processing oxygen and delivering it to the muscles, but there is a great deal more that goes into it. In fact, after a certain amount of aerobic exercise, we stop making gains in our heart health. We maximize the efficiency of the heart, and gains in our aerobic capacity have to come from other sources. Once we reach this point, we are no longer gaining any heart health benefits from the added aerobic exercise. Someone who runs marathons is not much less likely to have a heart attack than is someone who runs three miles, three times a week along with a regular resistance exercise program.

Having stated the above definitions, I will proceed to ignore them, as society as decided the word "cardio" encompasses the entire topic, as in "I'm going to do my cardio now." Aerobics has come to mean some sort of near dance like activity, done in unison following the instruction of an "Aerobics Instructor." So I'll use the work Cardio, semi-improperly for the rest of the book.

Why Cardio?

So having established that, we really need to define WHY we are doing cardio to determine how much is enough. If you simply love to run "ultra-marathons" then there probably isn't such a thing as "too much," as long as you are not suffering injuries that prevent you from competing. The competition is your "thing." It's what you enjoy, and as such, you should go for it.

Just don't fool yourself into thinking you're doing it for your health. Studies on just how much exercise is "enough" are lacking, and for very good reason, they are very difficult to conduct accurately and without being affected by other factors such as diet, smoking habits, etc. They also require a large number of study participants. The studies to date seem to indicate the greatest risk reduction from going from inactivity to some reasonable activity. The mortality curve seems to level off long before the range of aerobic capacity exhibited by competitive marathon runners.[19]

We ALL have some limit on the time we put into exercise, and I've found those who are overdoing the cardio are also the ones who are ignoring proper resistance training. Unless you are incorporating adequate resistance training, your quality of life as you age will probably also be less robust, especially considering the time you've put into exercising.

The fact is that much cardio is probably causing your body to tear down what it considers "unnecessary" bulk (muscle, bone, cartilage, tendons). Your body adapts to the stressors you put on it. If you continuously load your muscular-skeletal system to 10% of capacity (typical of most cardio), then your body thinks the other 90% is wasted capacity. You may have a healthy heart, but the rest of your body is deteriorating.

It is no coincidence that Dean Karnazes, perhaps the most successful ultra long distance athlete ever, is injury free and exhibits an all around musculature you won't see in most competitive long distance athletes. Dean doesn't just run, he mountain bikes, swims, rock climbs, windsurfs, and although he admits it's a last resort and bores him silly, hits the gym when necessary. In other words he has a well rounded program that works the entire body.

What if your goal is to lose weight (hopefully fat, not just weight). Well, cardio certainly does burn calories, but you have to run a long time to make up for even a small splurge in your diet. Snacking on bread at the restaurant before dinner might take over a half hour to burn off, and a jelly donut might take upwards of an hour of cardio to burn off.

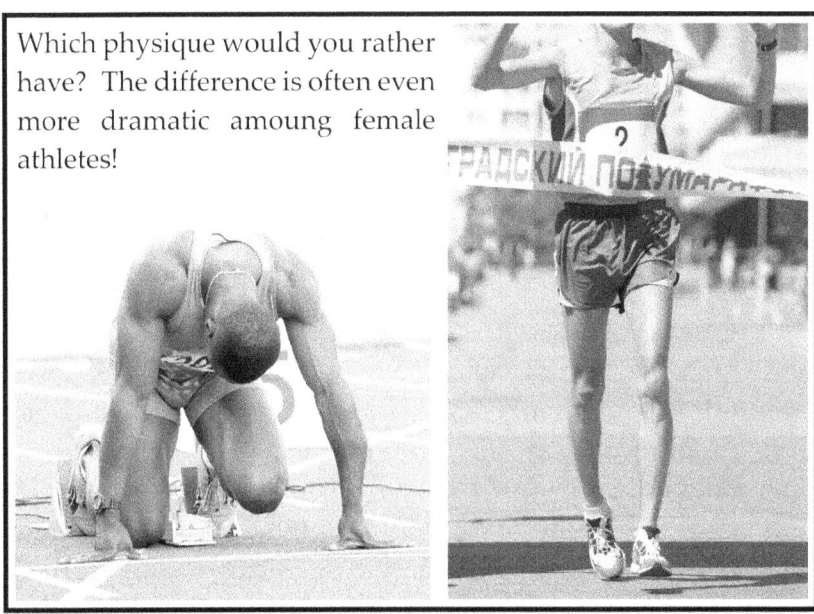

Which physique would you rather have? The difference is often even more dramatic amoung female athletes!

It's much easier to control your food intake in the first place, but if you simply love to eat, then endless hours of cardio may be your only answer. Just remember, at some point the more excessive your cardio is, the harder it will be to maintain or gain the lean muscle that makes us look "toned". Just compare the physique of a sprinter with that of a marathon runner. There's a reason you'll never see people like Richard Simmons or Jared from the Sub commercials without their shirt on!!!!

Now, if your goal is to look good, and be healthy, you need to make some compromises. Heart health is certainly VERY important. Everyone should get at least 20 minutes of cardio 3 times a week. Beyond that, my recommendation is to stick with the weights. In the long haul, resistance exercise will burn far more calories than cardio, and it will help you keep your precious muscle, even while dieting. We've all seen the anorexic girl that is nothing but skin and bones. Yes, she is thin, but no, she's neither healthy nor attractive.

If you're in a real hurry to lose as much weight as possible, or you just love to eat, and you're already doing 3 or 4 sessions of resistance exercise every week, then you can certainly up the cardio beyond the above recommendation. Remember, if you're trying to put on a little toned muscle, or you want to optimize your bodies "fat distribution patterns", more cardio isn't doing you any favors unless it's in the form of high intensity intervals (more on this later).

For sports performance, or simply for performance in the real world, you may need to up the time or intensity level of the cardio you are doing as well. You may have a healthy heart, but if your 15 year-old daughter is kicking your butt on the tennis court, running you into the ground, then you might want to think about stepping things up.

One of my main motivators for getting my indoor winter cardio in is that I know once I hit the mountain bike trails in the spring, I won't be enjoying the ride if I haven't been doing intervals on the exercycle during the cold months.

Types of Cardio

There are many ways to keep the heart healthy. In fact, if your resistance training uses short intervals, or circuits, you will be getting cardio in whether you know it or not, but for most goals, you'll need some sort of specialized cardio activity.

I'll divide cardio up based on intensity. Your body doesn't really care what actual activity you are doing as far as aerobic capacity is concerned (run, bike, swim, etc.), but the intensity level you use will drastically influence the results you are getting.

Low Intensity

This one is pretty easy to explain: get off the couch and take a walk. For individuals who are grossly out of shape, this may be the best overall form of exercise to start with. By starting slowly you reduce the risk of injury while still increasing your calorie expenditure. For many people, this is the most enjoyable form of cardiovascular exercise.

You can take your dog for a walk or spend some quality time with your spouse who also might use a break from the couch. You'd be amazed at what you might discover with a walk around your neighborhood. That old house you've driven by a 100 times at 40mph might fascinate you with its old style charm when you pass it at 3mph. You might even make some new friends. A slow bike ride also qualifies as low intensity cardio.

This type of cardio is also the form usually preferred by competitive bodybuilders who want to burn extra calories, but don't want to do ANY activity strenuous enough to interfere with their weight training. As a strength athlete AND mountain biker, I can attest to this one. Regardless of how hard I try to avoid it, every mountain bike season, my squat poundage's plummet. It's a compromise I'm willing to make, but to someone looking to put on as much muscle as possible the super high intensity activity of mountain biking is just too much.

There are reasons this low intensity cardio might not be the best for everyone. First is the fact that your overall cardio capacity will only improve so much without upping the intensity. You'll go a long way to preventing a heart attack, but don't expect to be able to keep up with your kids in a game of soccer because you've taken a few walks around the neighborhood.

Also, if you are using low intensity cardio to burn calories, plan on spending A LOT of time walking! One small dietary mistake (an average cookie), might take up to an hour to work off at a walking pace!!!

Medium Intensity

This is probably the most common form of cardio that most of you do. There is no definite line between low and medium intensity, but with medium intensity you will be working up a sweat. Running, fast biking, swimming, rollerblading, and race walking are all usually medium intensity cardio activities.

The advantages of medium intensity cardio include an increased calorie expenditure and higher cardiovascular capacity. A runner will burn far more calories in the same amount of time than a walker will. With medium intensity cardio, you will also find yourself getting into much better aerobic condition. That soccer game might not seem so tough after you can run a couple of nine-minute miles!

What are the disadvantages? First and foremost, BE CAREFULL!! If you are VERY out of shape, you should spend a couple months doing low intensity cardio before you move into medium intensity. Overexertion injuries as well as heart attacks and many other problems are possible in people who make the move to medium intensity too quickly. Even those of you who are not overweight, but have been sedentary for too long should start out slow.

Next, you also have to realize that medium intensity cardio is still not the ultimate weight loss solution. It's still going to take you a half hour to work off that cookie and your metabolism will still slow to normal immediately after this type of workout.

Also, don't think this type of activity will have you keeping up with Lance Armstrong on next year's Tour de France. Your aerobic capacity and anaerobic limit will only improve so much. Runners who are hitting performance walls, and amateur athletes in sports such as basketball, hockey, skiing, etc., will find huge benefits to moving to the next level of cardiovascular conditioning.

Medium intensity cardio (when used excessively) will also trigger the storage of intramuscular fat. (Think of a well-marbled piece of beef), as your body tries desperately to keep on hand the fuel needed for this type of workout. Excessive medium intensity cardio will also hinder muscle growth. Even if you are not trying to get big, muscle is still important for that "lean hard look".

Remember, your body is very good at adapting to the activities you are engaging in. Slow twitch muscle fibers with a lot of easily available fat stores for fuel is exactly what this type of activity requires. Not hard, strong, tight muscles like those of a gymnast or sprinter.

There is even some evidence that excessive medium intensity cardio might exaggerate lower body fat storage!!! Strangely enough, most women who are trying desperately to shrink their hips will do more and more medium intensity cardio ~ precisely the opposite of what they need!

High Intensity

This is the type of cardio that most of you should eventually be working towards. I often refer to this as "intervals". This consists of alternating bouts of very high intensity activity followed by very low intensity. An example on the stationary cycle: Warm up for 5 minutes at low intensity. Slowly increase the speed and or resistance until you reach a level that can only be maintained for 30 seconds. After 30 seconds, return to a slow light pace for 90 seconds. Repeat this pattern of 30 second sprints and 90 seconds at low intensity for 20 to 30 minutes total.

This is generally called HIIT or High Intensity Interval Training. Studies have shown it to burn up to three times as many calories as ordinary cardio.[20,21]

Following this protocol, you will have gotten the toughest cardio workout you've ever gotten, you'll have burned more calories than an hour of running, and you won't have triggered intramuscular fat storage (your muscles will be more like lean chicken than marbled beef). Most importantly for women not blessed with small lower proportions, you may even preferentially reduce lower body fat! You'll also minimize muscle loss since your body still gets the signal that it needs all the muscle it's got (the sprints were at near maximum capacity).

After a couple weeks of doing intervals, you'll also find you'll be able to do a lot more lifting in the weight room without losing your breath, and your work capacity in everyday life will show a huge improvement.

Intervals will improve both your anaerobic capacity as well as your aerobic capacity if you vary the duration of the intervals. A recent study also showed that adults that participate in interval type training maintained heart rate variability better than those who engaged in conventional steady state cardio. A decline in heart rate variability as we age has been associated with increased cardiovascular risk.[22],[23]

What are the disadvantages? Certainly, if you do not have a good base of fitness, you could really hurt yourself. I recommend moving up to this type of protocol slowly over time. In addition, this is not the most enjoyable form of exercise for many people. It's TOUGH, and you're not going to feel like making friends as you sprint around the neighborhood. Although depending on your dog, he may really enjoy some sprinting over the boring walk you usually take him on.

This type of cardio also has to be timed well to avoid hurting your leg workouts. I usually do this type of workout after a leg workout, or on an off day as long as I'm not working legs the next day. Although intervals of slightly less intensity (60sec. at 80 percent intensity instead of 30 at 100%) can be just as effective for most goals.

Some of the above advice may fly in the face of what you've been told in the past. Many people who are unclear on the basic concepts will talk about a "fat burning zone", and similar concepts. While it is true that lower intensity activity will burn a greater percentage of fat during the exercise than higher intensity activity, what these theories are missing is that the higher intensity activity still burns more calories overall, and that is what really counts. You don't really care when the fat calories were burned, just that more were burned. They all eventually result in body fat losses. As we discussed earlier, your body is very good at adapting to whatever stress you give it. If you are doing an activity that requires body fat, your body will attempt to compensate by storing more body fat for your next round of steady state cardio in the "fat burning zone."

GPP (General Physical Preparedness) Workouts

I know I initially said I was classifying types of cardio by intensity, but I feel I would be remiss without adding in GPP in a category of its own.

You'll remember I said earlier that one of the advantages of Intervals was that they pushed the limits of your energy systems? Well, there's another way to do intervals that will not only push your energy systems to new limits, but will also challenge your muscles in ways you never thought possible.

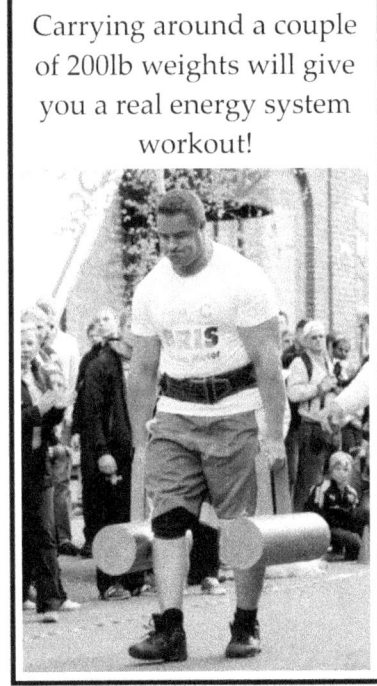

- The Farmers Walk -
Carrying around a couple of 200lb weights will give you a real energy system workout!

Conditioning coaches for strength athletes use these workouts because they drive the athletes to new levels of personal performance and cardio capacity without hampering muscle gains.

GPP workouts generally mimic some of the events you'll see in those "Worlds Strongest Man" competitions on ESPN. Sled dragging, rock carrying, truck pushing, etc. GPP workouts will make a man (or a strong woman) out of you. They are real world practical tasks. Not necessarily purely strength oriented like weight lifting, but requiring strength over a period of time.

This is a method of cardio that is certainly not for everyone, but if you think the concept sounds like more fun than sitting on an exercycle, then give it a try.

Some practical examples:

Farmers Walk: Pickup two heavy dumbbells and carry them around the gym. They should be heavy enough that you can't carry them for more than 30sec - 1 minute. Add some steps up and down off a step from the aerobics studio for an even better workout.

Sand Bag Carry: Do you have a backyard? Do you have a place to keep a couple 40lb bags of sand? Go out into the backyard and carry them around for a few minutes at a time.

Car Push: Do you have a car and driveway? Push and pull your car up and down the driveway.

Part of the fun and challenge of GPP is that it's so unorthodox, but that can also be a disadvantage, as not only may you not have access to the tools, but it's easier to hurt yourself than it would be working out in the gym. Take this into account and only attempt GPP if you're healthy and fit, and ready to take a few risks.

Calories Burned During Exercise

I hear it all the time: "I did the elliptical today and burned 1000 calories." People use the number on the machine to justify all sorts of bad dietary practice. Unfortunately, those numbers tend to be inaccurate. I've found various elliptical machines to be the worst offenders but all the machines are off to some extent.

Why would the companies do that? The answer is: to sell more machines. People tend to use the machines with which they can most easily burn the most calories. Gyms buy the machines people use the most. Personally, I feel this is the entire reason for the popularity of elliptical machines: they burn very few calories for the amount of motion going on (hence are actually not much of a workout), yet the indicated calories tend to be very high. You get the best (or worst) of both worlds: an easy workout that APPEARS to burn a lot of calories. In most gyms, the stairstepper machines tend to be the last to be used, yet this machine BY FAR provides the best workout, and best use of your cardio time.

It seems that virtually all machines tend to exaggerate a little bit, so I wouldn't trust any of them to justify that post workout ice cream sundae. If you want to get an idea of how many calories an activity will burn for a specific amount of time, try one of the calculators on the internet. There are several listed on my web site (www.thinkingpersonsfitness.com).

However even these calculators have three issues. First, they include BMR (Base Metabolic Rate) calories in the results. If it says you're burning 500 calories for a particular activity, but you would have burned 80 calories just sitting on the couch, then you really only burned 420 doing the activity. Including the BMR calories will cause you to basically double count the BMR calories.

Next, there is really no way to determine effort for many of the activities. It doesn't help that even with activities listed as so many "minutes per mile," it will still vary greatly per individual.

The third error in these calculations is the lack of accounting for post exercise energy expenditure. This is the amount of calories burned after you're done exercising. For running, biking or virtually any other steady state activity, this is virtually zero. For HIIT, weight lifting, or any other very high intensity activity, this can be up to three times the amount of the calories burned during the activity itself.

So, even though the calculator says you will only burn 300-500 calories in an hour of weight training, if you do it with enough intensity and are strong enough and experienced enough to lift some heavy weight, your total calorie burn over the course of 48 hours will be upwards of 1000-1500 calories.

I said earlier that you need to stop thinking about exercise in terms of "how many calories did I burn?". This is one of the reasons why. However, it is still important to understand this topic, if for no other reason than it reinforces the futility of worrying about how many calories a particular activity is burning.

When to do Cardio

There are many theories about when to do cardio: before your weight workout, after your weight workout, in the morning before breakfast, nighttime before bed, etc.

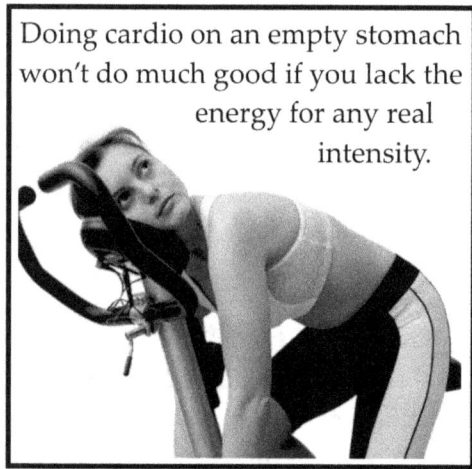

Doing cardio on an empty stomach won't do much good if you lack the energy for any real intensity.

The before breakfast crowd feels they'll burn more fat if they haven't eaten in a while. I can't say if that's true or not, as there are really no good studies, but just as with the "Fat Burning Zone" on the heart rate label on the machine, when it comes right down to it, it still only matters how many total calories you consume and how many total calories you use. It really doesn't matter if you burn body fat while you're exercising, if you're just going to put it right back on by eating more the rest of the day.

The two factors that should really affect your decision to do cardio on an empty stomach are as follows: first, can you get a good workout when you're body is in a fasted state? If the intensity of your workouts is suffering because you don't have the energy, then exercising on an empty stomach is probably a bad idea for you. The second factor is whether or not you'll just eat more the rest of the day to compensate. If you do your cardio on an empty stomach but then are SO hungry after your workout that you scarf down twice as much as you would otherwise, then all that fat is just being replaced anyway.

You have to remember that fat cells are like little gas tanks: burning fat doesn't destroy the fat cell. Once your body makes more fats cells, they're with you for life. Your body is very efficient at using the fat for fuel and then refilling the fat cells once you eat. It is very possible to do workouts that use very little fat for energy WHILE you're doing the workout, yet cause greater fat loss OVERALL.

As far as whether to do cardio on the same day as your resistance workout, well that's probably more a matter of convenience than anything. I imagine you'll probably get a better cardio workout (especially if it's intervals) on a separate day, but if you have a hard time getting to the gym extra days, and it's more convenient to have less trips that take longer, then I have no reason to tell you to do otherwise.

If you do your cardio on the same day as your resistance training, DEFINITELY do the resistance training first. You need the concentration and energy more for resistance training. If you're a little worn out for your cardio, it won't make near as much of a difference as if you were tired and lacked concentration for your weight training.

Some people like doing their cardio before bed. Personally, if I do cardio of any intensity anytime near my bedtime, there's no way I'm going to get to sleep, but that's an individual thing.

Don't put too much thought into when to do cardio. Do what is convenient for you, as that way you're much more likely to actually do it!

Chapter 8 – Essential Exercises

For the first few exercises in this chapter, maybe I could have titled it "Essential exercises you're NOT doing." I know I said this wasn't a book where I was going to describe every exercise, and I won't. But there are some exercises that are just too important not to cover how to do them and why they are so important.

Why am I sure most of you are not doing them? Because when I look around any gym, it's pretty obvious where everyone is spending their time, and it's not on these exercises.

Why are most of you not doing them? First, because they are tough. They put the "work" in working out. They require attention to do them correctly, and if done incorrectly, will result in injury rather quickly.

Some of these are exercises that work muscles you don't see in the mirror. But just because you don't check out your hams or your lats, doesn't mean others aren't.

It's no mystery why I'll start this chapter with exercises involving the legs. The biggest muscles in your body are in your legs. Working them can be just plain painful (in a good way). Most people will try virtually anything to get around working their legs the way they were meant to be worked:

- Machines that take all the stabilizing forces out of the very part of your body that need it most.
- Short range of motion exercises for muscles that so critically need adequate range of motion for quality of life and mobility.
- "Easier" exercises that never truly stress the muscles and bones of the very parts of our bodies that move us through our lives on a daily basis.

I'll talk more about posture in a later chapter, but it's no coincidence that we'll talk about some of the same exercises in that chapter as well. If you're not doing these exercises in some form, and doing them right, then chances are, you have bad posture.

Chances are also high that if you're not doing these exercises, you have problems maintaining your weight, and that you've noticed your metabolism decreasing as you age. These exercises are the "big" exercises that really hit all the big muscles. If you're not working those muscles correctly, not only are your workouts not burning as many calories as they could be, but your declining muscle mass is causing a drop in your metabolism as well.

Deadlifts

The hamstrings and sometimes the glutes (I hope it doesn't bother anyone that I'm not using the technically correct names), are probably the most neglected muscles in the body. In simple terms, the glutes are responsible for straightening your legs and the hamstrings have a dual role of both straightening the legs and bending the knees.

The glutes are sometimes trained by specific exercises which purport to target that area, usually in a vain attempt to spot reduce a flabby behind, but they are still often neglected.

The hamstrings are neglected even more. These muscles are really only heavily used in two circumstances, when you're sprinting, or when you're picking up something heavy with good form. Unfortunately, today, most of us do neither. Walking and distance running don't significantly activate the hamstrings, and no one sprints anywhere. Most people never lift anything heavy, and from watching the average person remove groceries from their trunk, I can conclusively say that very few people know how to lift with good form regardless of the load.

So if we never really use these muscles, why is it so important? Although we don't often work the hamstrings strenuously (and hence don't keep them strong), we do use them every day for posture. Weak hamstrings and glutes will result in bad posture as we'll talk about in a later chapter.

It's not just an appearance issue either. It's VERY complicated, and I won't even start to get into all of the interactions, but when weak hamstrings allow the pelvis to tilt, the spine and all its supporting musculature is compromised as well.

This leads us to the deadlift. As far as I'm concerned, the deadlift and its derivatives are the number one exercise for not only the hamstrings but also the glutes and the lower back. Most people work the hamstrings with leg curls (the hamstrings are a bi-articulate muscle, which means they pass through both the hip and knee joints), but unfortunately for a number of reasons, the leg curl won't do the job for these posture issues (although still a good exercise when used in conjunction with various forms of the deadlift).

Notice I keep saying "various forms of the deadlift"? That's because a true Deadlift is a very complicated exercise and probably shouldn't be attempted until you are an advanced lifter. One variation, the "Stiff Leg Deadlift", is much more effective at activating the hamstring, as well as being easier to do properly.

A deadlift is basically picking up a weight from the ground with perfect form (using the muscles of the legs and thighs, resulting in very low loads on the spine even at heavy weights). I'm not going to try to teach you how to do a true deadlift properly. It's a very complicated exercise that has several stages. Improper form in this exercise is sure to end in injury.

The stiff leg deadlift is the upper part of the conventional deadlift and doesn't utilize the quadriceps to bend the knees. A stiff leg deadlift looks a lot like someone bowing with a very straight back. The knees are kept slightly bent, but stiff. The lower back is slightly arched forward and this posture is maintained throughout the movement. Keeping the shoulders pulled back will help you maintain form throughout the movement. Lower the weight as far as you can while maintaining good form. Never compromise the arch of the lower back. If you round the lower back even slightly, the load on your spine will increase by a factor of five.[24]

A few more points: the deadlift works more muscles than just the hamstrings. Done properly the entire posterior chain is recruited. This exercise will burn MAJOR calories for days after the workout, and will hit the muscles of the lower back more effectively than any other "Core Workout".

The deadlift and its variants, aren't just an exercise, they're a teaching aid. Once you learn how to deadlift properly, you will have learned how to pick up anything properly. This is very important, because it's not necessarily the weight of the object you are trying to pickup that will hurt your back, but how you pick it up. Once this motion is ingrained in your muscle memory, you'll have a greatly reduced chance of hurting your back in the future.

Another way of working your glutes and hams is to incorporate sprints into your workout, but that's a topic for another section of the book.

So there you go. Find someone to teach you the stiff leg deadlift and start looking better (through better posture), feeling better (with a stronger lower back), and losing fat (because this exercise is so intense and uses so many muscle groups).

Stiff Leg Deadlift (SLDL)

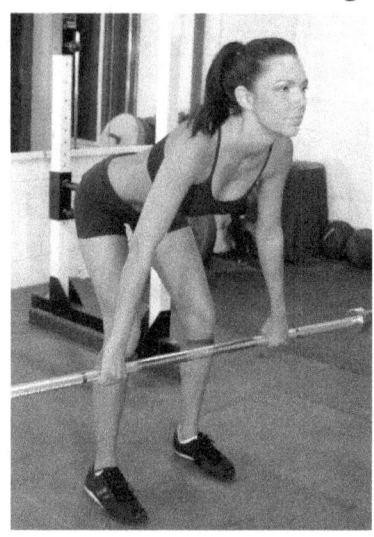

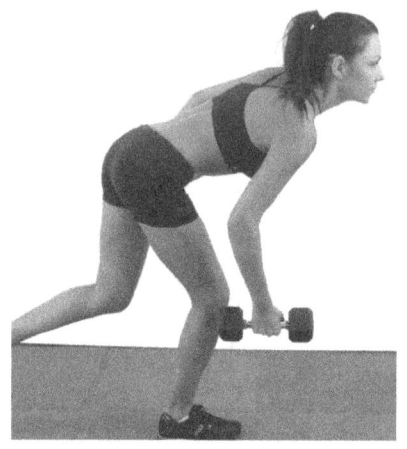

This is an easier to learn version of the deadlift, and for most people, just as useful.

The Single Leg Stiff Leg Deadlift is a little harder to master but a great addition to a normal SLDL.

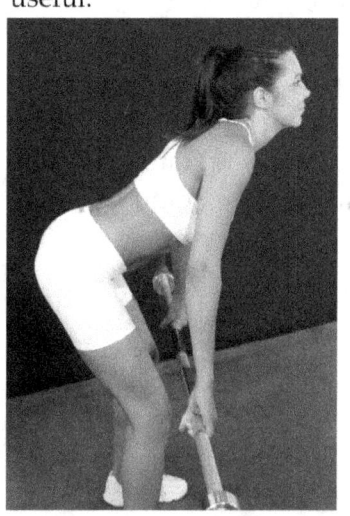

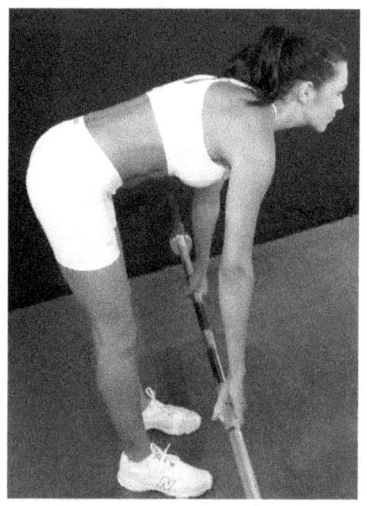

Notice the good arch in the photo on the left. The photo on the right is an exaggeration, but even a slight rounding of the back with cause lower back problems. The entire range of motion should be in the hips, NOT the lower back.

Squats

Yes, we've all heard it from some miss-informed expert at some point. "Don't do squats, they'll hurt your knees". I've personally heard more excuses for not doing proper squats in the gym than I could ever fit into this article: "I'm not built for squatting," "I've got long thighs," blah, blah, blah.

If you listen to the dogma, (20 years out of date dogma), squats will kill your knees, hurt your lower back, and are only done by big brutes attempting to bulk up.

Fortunately, that's not the case. Squats are the king all of exercises. Perhaps no other exercise works quite as many muscles in such a supremely functional manor. Think about it: what could be a more realistic and functional way of utilizing the human body than to use your legs and core muscles to lower and raise the upper body? It's an incredibly natural movement. Babies do it before they can walk, and people of ALL ages do it as part of everyday life in other cultures!

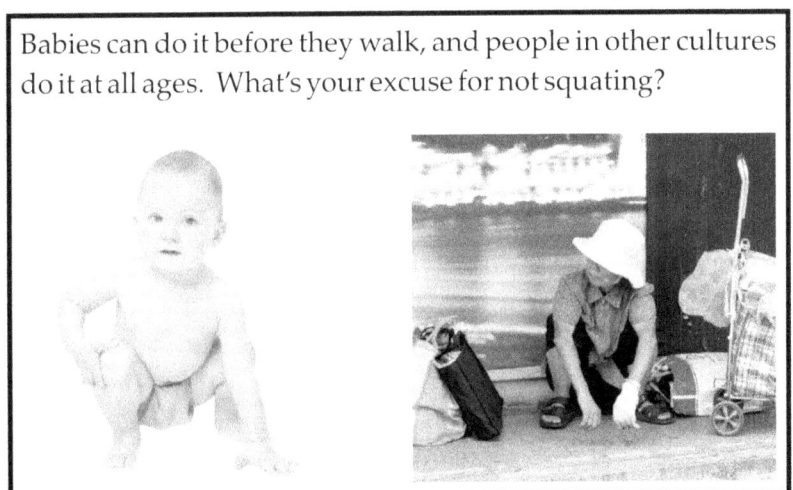

Babies can do it before they walk, and people in other cultures do it at all ages. What's your excuse for not squating?

Hard core exercise gurus have a saying: "If you're not squatting, you ain't doing squat." Cliché, yes, but true. Although there are many other exercises that work the same muscles in smaller groups, no other exercise hits so many muscles so well.

Squat's will not make you bulky: eating too much or doing steroids can make you bulky, but unless you're a genetic mutant, doing a couple sets of squats with your workout will keep your legs strong, fit and toned, and help burn A LOT of calories! They're not just for guys!

When done properly, squats do not hurt the lower back. Just as with deadlifts, not allowing the lower back to round even slightly is the key. When posture is maintained throughout the lift, the chances of injuring your back are less than doing many daily functions like lifting a bag of groceries incorrectly.

Squats are also much better for the knees than other more common exercises such as leg extensions. In fact, I religiously recommend squats for my clients who are amateur athletes dealing with knee problems. As long as there is no existing structural issue that needs a surgeon's attention, the strengthening effect of squats on ALL the muscles that support the knee will almost always result in improvement and pain reduction.

On several occasions, I've worked with amateur athletes with knee problems. Other "experts" had told them to stop squatting; nevertheless, their knee problems worsened over the years. After getting these same clients back "under the bar" for a few months, their knee problems vanished.

The squat is also more than just a single exercise. By varying the stance and bar location, this exercise can work the quadriceps, hamstrings, abductors, adductors, glutes, lower back muscles, abs, and many other muscles too numerous to mention. Jump squats, box squat, band squats, back squats, front squats, etc., however you utilize them, squats should be the core of your leg workouts!

By varying the stance from wide to medium to narrow from workout to workout, you can completely change the function of this exercise and you'll really feel it in different parts of your legs.

- Wide stance: By positioning the feet much wider than shoulder width, the hamstrings take over much of the work the quads would normally perform, and the abductors are hit harder. I'll go as wide as the edge of the rack to really hit the hams and abductors.
- Narrow stance: Bring the feet in to just under the shoulders and the quads dominate. You really feel it in the adductors. Some people find it hard to go low enough with a narrow stance, while others will go as narrow as a couple inches apart.

Along with feet position, you can also change it up with how you hold the bar. There are quite a few bar position options, but the two most important are front and back squats. These two seem to work various muscles differently in different people. I'm sure it has a lot to do with leg and torso lengths, but all you need to know is that by changing how you hold the bar, you will fundamentally change the exercise. Don't be afraid to experiment.

Wide, Narrow, and Front Squat Variations

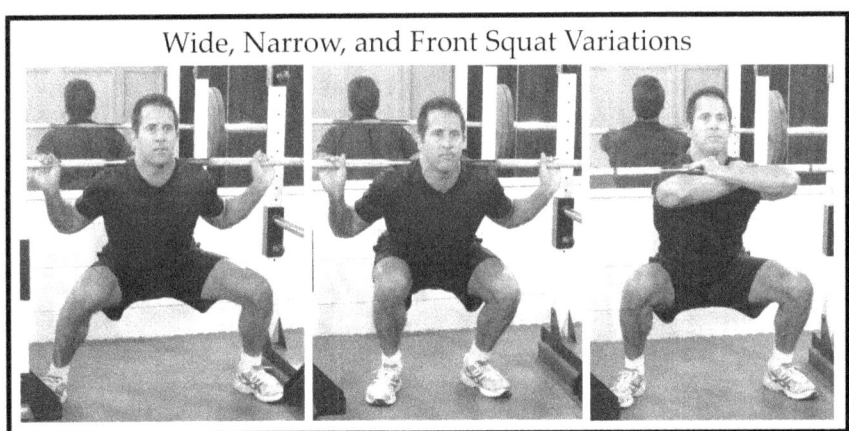

Here's the big problem: If not done properly, you can hurt yourself VERY quickly. Form is of utmost importance. What is most disconcerting to me is that I rarely see anyone actually performing this exercise correctly.

The difference between good form and bad form can be subtle to the eyes, but not for your lower back. The difference is 5 to 10 times as much shear load on the spine when using the posture on the right!!

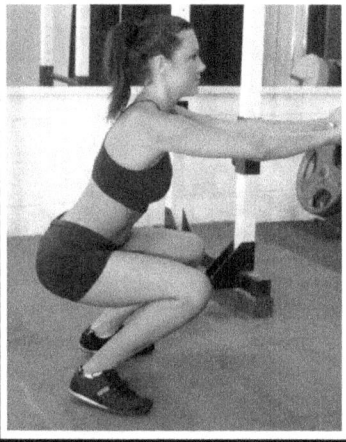 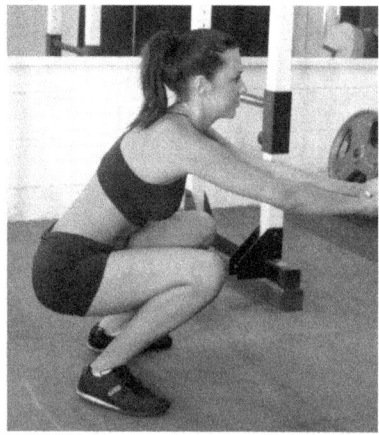

The following hints will help you to get started, but I would highly recommend seeking additional assistance from someone who knows what they're doing, and can personally instruct you on proper form.

1. Start off without any weight at all. Your feet should be slightly wider than shoulder width apart and your toes may point slightly outward if this is more comfortable for you. Concentrate on sitting down, not bending forward.

You should be able to do a deep knee bend to where your hips are even with your knees. Make sure you can do 20 of these without pain before moving on to a weighted squat. Your heels should stay on the ground. If you can't seem to keep your heels on the ground all the way down, you may need to stretch the soleus muscles in the back of your legs. You can do this by performing any standard calf stretch with your knees bent.

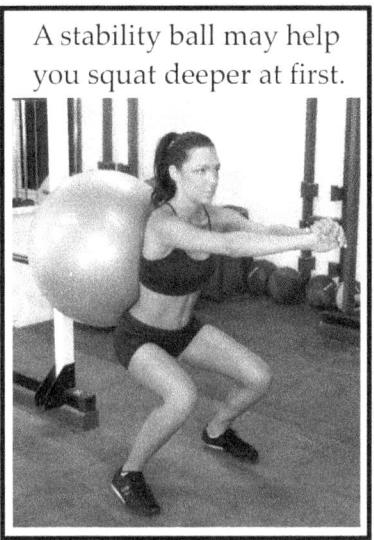

A stability ball may help you squat deeper at first.

If you have trouble with the unweighted squats because your knees are particularly bad, it may be helpful to start off by leaning against a stability ball.

2. Once you are comfortable with unweighted squats you'll want to move on to dumbbells. Maybe just some five pounders to start. Move up in weight when you can do 15 reps. Your back should stay flat. Watch this in a mirror from the side. Never let your back round! When the muscles that support your core are holding your back flat (spine neutral), there is almost no load on the spine itself. As soon as you round your back, the load on your spine increases dramatically.

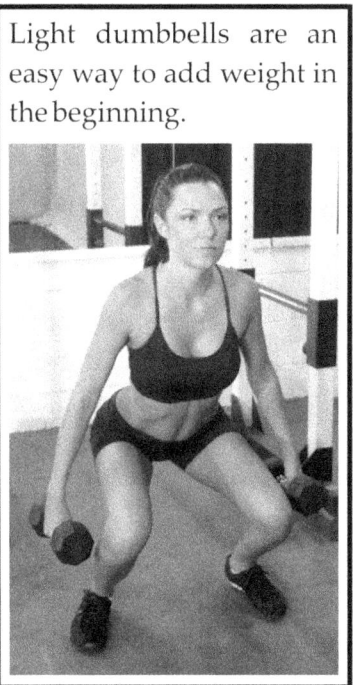

Light dumbbells are an easy way to add weight in the beginning.

3. Once you move up to 15 or 20lbs in each hand, you may find it easier to switch over to working with a barbell.

- Position an empty bar on the rack at a height that allows you to lift it off the rack without standing on your toes.
- Squat under the bar with your feet firmly under the bar. The bar should be positioned comfortably on

the muscles of your shoulder, not resting against your spine. A Manta Ray may help with this (go to the product section of www.thinkingpersonsfitness.com).

- Lift the bar from the rack and step slowly away from the supports. Make sure your feet are the proper width apart and your toes pointed forward or slightly to the side. Tense your midsection (don't suck it in). This will form a natural weight belt and properly support your spine. DON'T use a real weight belt. Yes, it may help support your lower back, but in the process, it will rob you of a valuable core workout, and help assure you of injuring your lower back in the real world. The squat is one of the best core exercises you can do since it utilizes the muscles of the midsection and posterior chain the way they were supposed to be used (to stabilize the spine under load). Don't sacrifice this by using a belt.

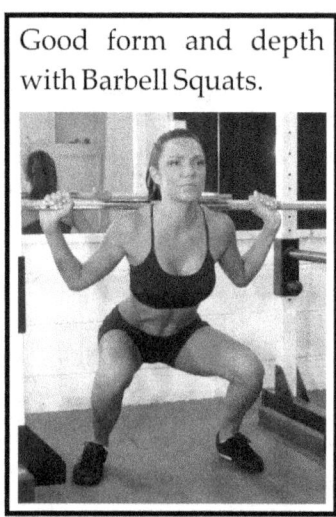

Good form and depth with Barbell Squats.

- Now squat down. Concentrate on sitting down and lowering your rear end, not lowering the bar. The bar will come down naturally. If you watch yourself in a mirror, your hips should come down to at least even with your knees. The tops of your thighs should be parallel with the ground. If you can't come down that far, decrease the weight. This isn't an ego contest. It doesn't matter how much weight you can use.

Now it's time to dispel a myth: "Never let your knees pass over your toes." While it's true that the further your knees extend over your toes the higher the load on this joint, the fact is the increase in load with proper form is not significant.[25] For the vast majority of people, keeping their toes behind their knees will result in an improper arch of the lower back, causing the load on the spine to massively increase. Powerlifters can keep their knees behind their toes because their naturally short upper legs and the huge amounts of weight they are lifting, (several times their own body weight), allows them to balance this way. This won't be the case for most of you.

Regardless of your goals, squats should always play a role in your workouts.

Horizontal Pulling – Rows

This is the most overlooked or underutilized exercise for the upper body. Seems everyone wants to do horizontal pushing exercises (bench press) but very few care about pulling. That's ironic because the very reason most people bench press (bigger, firmer chest) is precisely the look you will get from the opposite movement - rows.

Trying to add any significant size to the pecs is hard. As strange as it sounds, it's a strong upper back coupled with a properly stretched chest that will show off the upper front of your physique. This is true for both men and women. More on this in the section on posture.

There are more ways to row than perhaps any other exercise. I highly recommend trying as many as possible. It's hard to go wrong with rows as long as you are doing them. Very few people injure themselves rowing other than those that let their back round during the exercise.

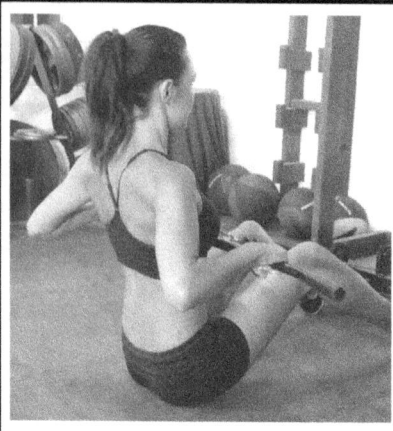

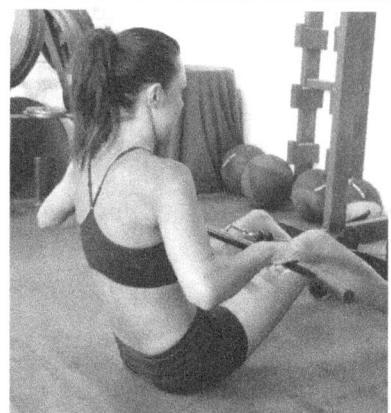

Top Left - Seated Row with good form.

Top Right - Seated Row with bad form.

Bottom Right - Bent over row with good form.

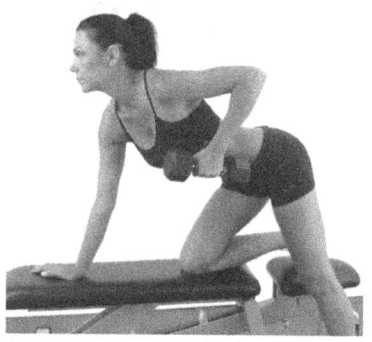

Horizontal Pushing – Bench Press

This is not one of the overlooked exercises. Pretty much everyone uses some form of these, and they are necessary, as long as you don't overdo it or use bad form. Don't lift with your ego (go too heavy), and do experiment with different variations of this exercise.

I personally prefer dumbbell bench presses, as they are easier on the shoulders (less chance of rotator cuff injuries over time), and a recent informal study showed they actually hit the various muscles better then the barbell version.[26] The closer you pull your arms into your body, the more you will be working the back of your arms (triceps) and the further out your arms are, the more you will work your shoulders and chest.

Vertical Pulling – pull-ups, chin-ups

These exercises are necessary to work the muscles of the middle of your back. No one ever seems to be able to explain why, but pull-ups and chin-ups seem to work better than pull-downs with a bar and cable, but many of you won't be able to pull up your entire body weight at the beginning, so using the cable machine is fine.

Varying the grip will change the muscles this exercise is hitting. A palms forward grip (pull-up) will hit the back more, whereas a palms facing you grip (chin-up) will hit the arms more. A wider grip will also hit the back more than the arms, and make the exercise tougher at the same weight as well. Experiment with different grips often.

Some people will pull the bar down behind the neck. If you have VERY good shoulder mobility, this MAY activate the lats a little better than pulling the bar down in front, but it is generally unnecessary and potentially hazardous to shoulder health.

Vertical Pushing – Military press

This exercise works the top of your shoulders and the backs of your arms. Unless you're a professional bodybuilder, forget about all of the various shoulder exercises like upright rows and shrugs, various versions of the Military Press will probably be all you'll ever need for your shoulders.

Just make sure to use good form, and adjust your arm position and the depth to which you lower the weight to avoid any pain in the shoulders. DO NOT work through the pain. Once you mess up your shoulders, you'll be struggling with the pain for the rest of your life.

For this reason, I don't recommend behind the head shoulder presses. Like behind the neck pull-downs, some people can do them without issues, but most simply do not have the functional range of motion to lower the weight behind their head. It's not a matter of stretching either. That motion is simply not natural for most. The human shoulder was not designed to press backwards.

Final Exercise Notes

One last word on form: proper form is crucial in all exercises! Keeping the lower back neutral or slightly arched will go a long way to helping you to stay free of lower back injuries. At the start of virtually all exercises, the muscles of your core should be "braced" like a boxer preparing to get hit. Do not "suck it in". Instead, simply tense all of the muscles in and around your stomach and lower back.

The same moderate but constant tensing of this boxers abdominal muscles are what will also protect you from lower back injuries both in the gym and out.

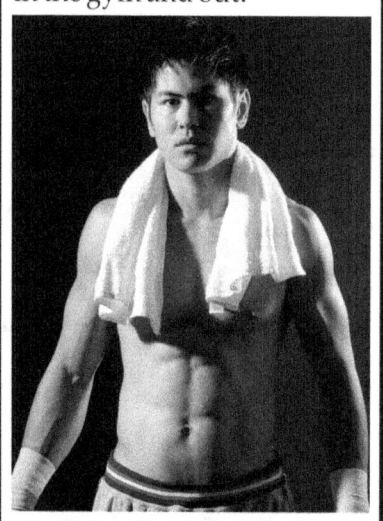

Do not do any movement that causes pain. Discomfort is a standard part of working out, but if anything seems to cause pain in a joint, stop immediately and find a way around the pain. Every person is different, and a movement that others can do with ease, may not be natural for you. Varying hand and foot positions to help you find a way that is comfortable for you, will help you avoid pattern overload injuries as your years in the gym add up.

Chapter 9 – Samples Workout

I do not want this book to be about showing you exactly how to work out. I want it to be about learning how to work out so you can make your own decisions and setup workouts that work best for you and your goals. This book is intended for the "thinker" who knows he needs to understand what he is doing, because he or she is an individual.

However, you do need somewhere to start. You can find more workouts on my web site, and I encourage you to sign up for my monthly newsletter where I will be sending out workouts and other updated information. Six years of my newsletter is how this book got started, so if you like what you're reading now, you'll also like the information in the free newsletter.

Your First Workout

To show you just how simple it should be, I'll give you an example of a workout I put almost every client on for the first month or so. Yes, I said almost every client! I know I've said throughout this book that everyone is different, but the core of the program works for almost everyone.

First, it teaches the basic lifts that you will use throughout all your future workouts. If you don't find yourself coming back to these core lifts, you're probably suffering for it.

Next, these basic lifts will hit just about every muscle in the body and, if programmed the way I recommend, will start to correct any imbalances. If you have a particular dislike for any of these exercises, that's probably the one you need the most. If it were easy, it wouldn't be a workout.

For the basic workout, you'll be doing three full body workouts per week. You'll also be doing basic cardio as described in that section. If getting to the gym is a hassle, take a little extra time and do the cardio on the same days, but if you can, do your cardio on separate days.

The workout itself should take no longer than 45 minutes. Count on adding 5 minutes up front to warm up, and if you don't like doing your stretching between sets, add some time on the end for stretching.

Your workout will use six different exercises: a quad dominant leg exercise, a hamstring dominant leg exercise, a horizontal pushing exercise, a horizontal pulling exercise, a vertical pushing exercise, and a vertical pulling exercise.

For your first couple of weeks, or until you get the hang of the basics, you'll be using the following exercises: Squat, Stiff Leg (straight back) Deadlift, Bench Press, Row, Military Press, and Pull down.

You will start out with three "supersets" of two exercises. For this program, they will always be unrelated exercises. For your first time through, you'll do two sets of each exercise. If you make it through this easily, you can move up to three sets of each exercise. At that point, your workout will look like this:

1A. Squat
1B. Bench Press
2A. SL Deadlift
2B. Row
3A. Military Press
3B. Pull Down

The notation "1A, 2A, etc." is the commonly used notation for supersets. In this case, you would do a set of squats, and set of bench presses, then another set of squats and another set of bench presses. So, for your first workout, you would do a total of 12 sets. For your second workout you would do 18 sets (three of each superset).

You should start out doing easy sets of 16 to 18 reps for the first few workouts until you learn the exercises. After you get the hang of the exercises, add weight anytime you can do more than 14 reps. The first two sets of each exercise should not be to failure. After you gain some experience, the last set should be to failure or beyond (forced reps if you have a spotter). With more experience (after a month or so) work in a higher weight/ lower rep range (10-12), but be especially careful that your form is good.

After several workouts (I can't tell you how many. It will differ for everyone), you'll probably find that 18 sets go by in less than 45 minutes and you'll feel like you could have done more. At that point, you can add sets at the end. Pick an exercise for a body part that you really want to work on. You might want to add some swiss ball crunches for your abs, calf raises or some curls for your biceps. In this way, you'll be customizing the workout as you go along.

You'll probably make steady progress with this routine for many months. At the start, you will gain strength, but not see much in the way of appearance. Don't worry, it will come.

At some point, you'll start getting bored or your results will slow. Once this happens, you can start to choose alternative exercises for each category.

Leg - Quad Dominant*	Leg - Ham Dominant*
Squat	SL Deadlift
Lunge	DeadLift
One Leg Squat	Leg Curl
Split Squat	Single Leg SLDL
Leg Extension	
Push - Horizontal	Push – Vertical
Bench Press (db or bb)	Military Press
Incline Press (db or bb)	One Arm Military
Push-up	Handstand push-up
Pull - Horizontal	Pull – Lower Back
Seated Row	Pull-Down (Pronated grip)
Bent over Row	Chin-Down (Supinated grip)
One Arm Bent Row	Pull-Up or Chin-Up

* Almost all of the leg exercises will hit both the quads and hams. Some that are considered quad dominant might be ham dominant in certain individuals. Don't worry about it too much. As long as you are doing a variety of these exercises, you'll hit all the muscles of your legs.

Make sure to return to the core exercises at least once a week, and keep track of the weight and reps you can do on these exercises. You should keep improving on the core exercises even though you are only doing them once per week. If you are not, something is wrong. Take a step back and make sure you're really doing what you should be doing.

As you learn more exercises, you can substitute them for the ones in the chart. Just make sure the basic pattern is there. You don't want to end up neglecting certain muscles. If you're not paying attention, you'll probably end up neglecting the back side of your legs (hamstrings and glutes) and your upper back. No coincidence that they happen to be muscles you can't see in the mirror.

Once you reach a certain point, you'll want to experiment with various rep ranges. The general rule of thumb for experienced lifters is that 1-8 reps is good for strength, 8-12 reps is best for building muscle, and 12- is for muscle endurance. This is just a rule of thumb, as it will vary not only from individual, but also will change depending on the part of the body you are training. For most people, the 8-12 rep range is also the range that works best for weight loss.

If you learn how to customize this workout intelligently, it can take you a long way. For most people, it may be all you need. If you want to put on a little more muscle rather than just being "fit," you might want to get a little more complicated.

There you have it. A simple, but customizable starter program. I know, it's not near as glamorous as some of the programs you see in the magazines, but that's the point. It gets the job done in the minimum amount of time. More complicated is NOT necessarily better! Remember KISS!

Stepping It Up

If you've spent some time on this starter routine, but you've decided you want to take it to the next level. Maybe because your results have slowed down with the starter routine, and you're looking for a level of fitness that gets LOOKS, with a musculature that stands out. At that point, you'll need to step it up.

If your goals do go beyond what you can achieve with full body workouts, you'll need to hit the weight room at least 4 or 5 days a week, and at that point, a split routine makes sense. You'll also be hitting each muscle harder in each workout, so you can work each part of your body a little less often, but at the expense of some added soreness at times.

You can split your workouts up as simply as the common upper and lower body split, or you can get far more complicated. The more complicated you get the harder you must make each workout. If you've split the body into four parts, and you're only doing four resistance training sessions per week, then you've got an entire week for that body part to recover: you better have really blasted every muscle in each workout or you'll be backsliding between workouts.

One of the splits I use most often relies on the fact that I abuse my legs pretty badly with either high intensity intervals, plyometrics or sports. I'll do upper body push, lower body , and upper body pull days in the weight room, then a separate day of HIIT, plyometrics, sports or a combination of them. I find I get so much lower body work from jumping, sprinting, or cranking up a hill on my mountain bike that I find I really can't use more than one day out of three on legs.

How often you workout will depend to large extent on how hard your workouts are and how well your body recovers.

Someone with great recovery ability (young and healthy) may do:

Day 1 – Upper Body Pull
Day 2 – Lower Body
Day 3 – Upper Body Push
Day 4 – Intervals and Plyometrics
Day 5 – Off
Day 6 – Start Over with Upper Body Pull

Someone with slower recovery might be better off with:

Day 1 – Upper Body Pull
Day 2 – Lower Body
Day 3 – Off
Day 4 – Upper Body Push
Day 5 – Intervals and Plyometrics
Day 6 – Off
Day 7 – Start Over with Upper Body Pull

This is where I'm going to leave it to other sources. You can hardly pickup a fitness magazine without another new "best ever" workout split. I'm sure you can get plenty of ideas from them or my web site (www.thinkingpersonsfitness.com) where I'll periodically put up a new workout for a specific goal. Just make sure you're sticking to the basics of workout construction that I presented earlier.

Chapter 10 – Working Out for Sports

Although I've always known how effective a good resistance training program can be for an athlete of any level, I have still been surprised at how many of my clients have told me what a tremendous improvement their performance in their sport of choice has shown since starting my program.

Although many sport training "gurus" will tell you that you need a highly specialized training program just for your sport, the actual truth is that trying to tailor the program around the dynamics of your particular sport will only result in more injuries and muscle imbalances. In fact, what most amateur athletes really need is a good "whole body" conditioning program with some small modifications for the specifics of each sport.

What are we looking to accomplish in the gym if we are looking for improved sports performance? First, you have to realize that you are not doing sports training in the gym any more than a professional athlete is. Both the professional and the amateur should separate their sports training from their strength and conditioning training.

Your strength and conditioning training WILL improve your sports performance, but only because it improves your body's overall conditioning, not because it improves any sport specific skill or movement.

If you try to mimic the sport in question in the gym, you will not do it well. Whether it's the environment or the implements, your movements will be off, and you'll end up hurting the real movement. You'll also further overuse (abuse) the muscles and joints that you are already overusing in the sport. Examples of this would be trying to mimic a golf swing with a weighted club or trying to duplicate a throwing motion on a machine.

The specific attributes that you can improve in the gym that will help you on the court or field are:

- Overall strength
- Functional range of motion
- Prehab (injury proofing your body)
- Stamina
- Rehab (recovering from an injury)

The best way to do this is with a basic resistance training and interval cardio program that works ALL the muscles of the body. With a properly designed program, the weaker muscles will eventually be brought up to the level of the stronger ones. The program should also include a variety of compound unilateral and twisting movements (movements that work each side of the body separately) or involve twisting of the torso in a controlled manner.

Professional athletes with professional strength and conditioning experts MAY be able to create custom tailored programs by working with the sporting coach to come up with specialized training programs to build up an athlete's weak areas. But you are probably not a professional athlete, and any coach you hire is probably also training 100 other people and doesn't really have time to figure out your particular issues. Besides, you're looking for improvements of 10-20% (easy to achieve with a proper conditioning program) whereas a pro athlete has already found that 10-20% and is looking for a 1% (or less) improvement in their game.

The truth is you are probably going to be better off with a general program such as the one outlined previously, than you will be with any trainer who purports to "specialize" in amateur athletes.

Be VERY wary of programs offering "balance" or "stability" training as I stated earlier. Those programs will over use unstable surfaces such as balance boards and balls. Although these devices can be useful at times, the proprieceptors in your muscles should be trained to work WITH your inner ear and eyes to provide balance and stability, not against each other. Training on an unstable surface will only help you if the sport you are playing is on an unstable surface. One example would be using a balance board at home if you are a snowboarder but can't always get to the slope (check out the Bongo Board in the Products section of my site).

Don't underestimate the value of weight loss either! Although we've all seen examples of pro athletes that were a little pudgy and still excellent at their sport, the fact remains that if you're hauling around an extra 20-40 lbs it WILL affect your game. You'll be surprised at how your reaction times and endurance will improve if you get your body fat down. Of course, you MUST lose the weight the right way. If all you do is starve yourself, or spend endless hours on the treadmill, you'll lose almost as much muscle as fat, and that definitely won't help your performance.

You will often hear old fashioned dogma such as "You can't lift if you're going to (Pitch, play golf, run fast, etc., etc). I'm amazed at how many people still think working with weights will make you stiff and muscle bound. It just isn't so. Yes, if you're trying to set personal records in the bench press the day before you hit the links, your game will undoubtedly suffer, but if you do it right, resistance training will only help your game.

Although a general, well planned conditioning program may be all you need for your sport, the following will give some specific hints for some of the more common sports in which my clients have participated in.

Golf

The thought that anyone would spend time in the gym in order to become a better golfer used to be almost laughable to most people. While some of us have known for years that just about any sport can benefit from a proper conditioning program, it took pros like Tiger Woods to finally bring it to the mainstream. Now no one doubts the benefits a proper conditioning program can provide for your golf game.

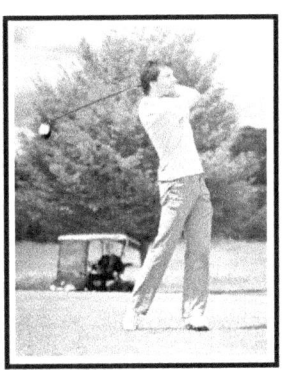

The most common improvements my clients see are: longer drives with less effort, the ability to play longer (more holes) without a fall-off in their scores (due to fatigue), no reoccurrence of injuries or specific muscle soreness that had bothered them in past years.

In my opinion, joint strength and integrity is at the top of the list when training for golf. By improving the strength and stability of the muscles, tendons and ligaments that control each, you can greatly improve your swing, and condition those joints to resist fatigue and injury.

To do this we don't necessarily utilize movements that mimic the golf swing. In fact quite the contrary, those motions get plenty of work on the course. What we really need to do is strengthen all the muscles that control the joints, but aren't really the prime movers in the swing itself. Those are the muscles that are weak from years of playing, and therefore will contribute to injury. They are also probably the muscles which are causing your swing to be less controlled and powerful than you'd like.

The next important factor is adequate, but properly controlled range of motion. Many trainers think this involves long sessions of static stretching. Unfortunately, this can be counterproductive in many instances. Studies show that too much static stretching will lengthen the ligaments and tendons that control the joints. This will increase your range of motion, but at the expense of control of the joints motion. This will result in increased risk of injury, as well as a DECREASE in control of the swing. What I recommend is a moderate amount of static stretching, as well as resistance training that emphasizes a full range of motion. The only way to train a muscle to function properly through its full range of motion (as in Golf) is to train it through the full range of motion. Studies have conclusively shown that a muscle will only adapt in a range of 10 degrees of where it's worked. By training all the muscles of the body through full range of motion exercises, you allow the joints to adapt to functioning properly through that full range of flexibility.

To summarize, beware of golf conditioning programs that simply try to copy the golf swing in the gym. If you wanted to swing the club some more, you'd just go to the driving range. If you really want to improve your game, stick to the basics. It is very common for my clients to improve their handicap more through six months of a conventional fitness program than they have in the last ten years of working on their game itself.

Racket Sports

Much of what I said in the previous section applies to Tennis and Racquetball as well. Keeping the shoulders, elbows, and wrists strong and functionally flexible is critical to injury prevention.

Interval training is a "must do" for racket sports. You're

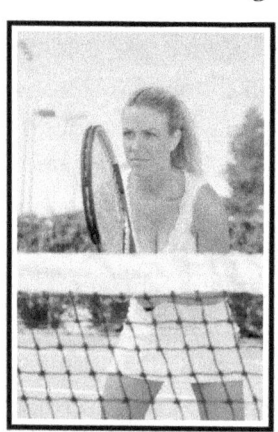

never at a steady state during a game so why train that way by doing steady state, low intensity cardio. Any single volley may last ten seconds to a minute at most and during that time, you'll be moving at near maximum effort. This is precisely what HIIT will train you for.

Don't underestimate the value of squats and deadlifts for racket sports. Strong legs are essential for moving your body around quickly.

Snow Skiing or Snowboarding

Muscle endurance is the name of the game for snow sports. Everything stated in the opening section applies, but endurance plays an even more important role.

Most of us don't go skiing one day a week, every week. Most of us go on ski trips where we go at it for 5 days straight. If you want to really enjoy the trip and get maximum vertical, you need to have some serious muscular endurance.

What I've found to be most helpful is to use conventional rep ranges on your leg training COMBINED with high intensity cardio training on a stairstepper (preferred) or exercycle. Unlike tennis where a play is always less than a minute, most skiing will involve your legs taking a beating 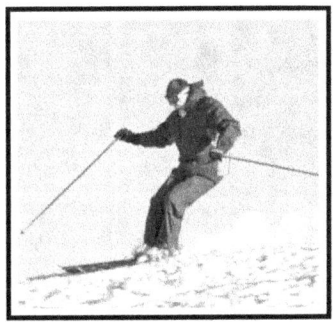 for several minutes at a time. As such, training intervals should be more on the order of 2-5 minutes (Maybe we could call this MIIT or Medium Intensity Interval Training). Go at an intensity such that you can't go any further at the end of each interval. When trying to get back into the season, I will often train legs by separating each resistance set with one interval on the stairstepper. My cardio days will consist of multiple 3 minute intervals. I'll even stick a couple of stairstepper intervals in with my upper body days. The trick here is to teach your body that it's not going to get a break. It needs to learn to recover FAST.

Making your legs and core stronger in general will help a lot, especially at the beginning. When you first start strength training your legs are probably not nearly strong enough. Yes, skiing isn't a sport of maximum strength for the pros as they are probably using 30-40% of their maximum strength, but in the beginning, you won't be nearly as strong, and certain moves on the mountain may push you to near 100%. This will wear you out much faster, as well as slow down your reaction time a lot.

Get stronger through a variety of bilateral AND unilateral leg training, and your reaction and endurance will improve.

Running

As with golf, ten years ago all anyone thought you had to do to train for endurance sports was do the sport. If you wanted to run a marathon, run more.

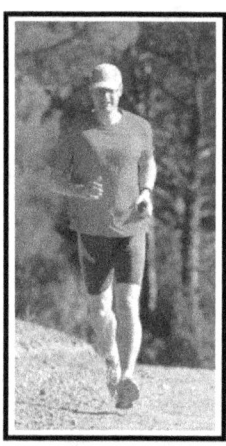

Today, most endurance trainers recommend a combination of training that includes intervals as well as some time in the gym. Although you may not want to put on muscle (not likely if you're running 80 miles per week), resistance training or at least cross training, will greatly improve your resistance to injury and extend your career in the sport.

I won't spend any more time on this topic as there are other much more knowledgeable endurance sport trainers.

Biking

For biking, leg strength usually takes a back seat to lower body endurance. Although I won't disagree with that, I do feel

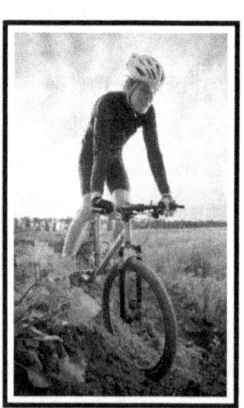

lower body strength training can really help. The stronger you are, the lower the percent of your max effort you will be using, and I've found that to be an advantage. Especially for Mountain Biking where you will often find yourself grinding up a steep hill at a very low cadence, having strong legs will really help.

Upper body strength will also help in Mountain biking, where you'll often be throwing yourself and your bike around technical sections. The more effort you have to expend on your upper body, the less you'll have to pedal. Having a little extra upper body strength makes the tough sections seem a lot easier.

One of the problems with resistance training alongside biking is that you have to time your workouts carefully. It's easy to ruin a good ride by overworking your legs in the gym the day before. You'll either need to time your leg workouts carefully or keep them short.

If I haven't included your specific sport here, don't let that stop you. They're just the most common ones my clients participate in. Just getting in shape in general will help your game dramatically, regardless of what sport you play.

Chapter 11 – Injuries

"I will endure the pain that goes with achievement and glory, rather than accept the contentment that goes with mediocrity."

Whether you're an athlete, or sit on the couch all day, injuries are a part of life. The athlete, amateur or professional, who goes their entire career without an injury, is rare. Those that do are both lucky and smart. The couch potato will probably end up with a bad back, sore knees, hips, etc.

I'd love to be able to say that injuries should never happen in the gym. If you're playing sports, they may be unavoidable, but in the controlled environment of the weight room or cardio equipment, shouldn't proper form and programming pretty much eliminate injuries?

Perhaps, but in my experience, from time to time, even the most careful exerciser will suffer from an injury or two. Avoiding injuries in the first place is certainly the best strategy, but given that sometimes bad things happen to good people, how you deal with your injuries is equally important.

Good Pain - Bad Pain

You've heard all the quotes. If you're a professional athlete, there are times you are expected to endure physical pain that will cause permanent damage to your body: "play through the pain."

But you're not a professional athlete. The object here is to build your body up over time, not tear it down. At the same time, I've had far too many clients that thought any discomfort was a reason to take time off. If you're over 16, you should have figured out by now that any goal worth achieving will require some discomfort. The hard part is figuring out the difference between possibly debilitating pain, and discomfort.

If you are working out with any intensity at all, there will be times when a particular part of your body will be sore. Sometimes this is just the soreness that goes along with working out, but sometimes it's the start of something serious.

Sometimes injuries are sudden and obvious. Drop a 45lb plate on your toes, and the crunch that you hear will tell you what you need to know even before the pain hits. Let your ego talk you into getting into a bench press competition with that big guy at the gym, and the "pop" you hear in your chest as you try to bench way more than you should, along with the huge bruise that develops over the next day will let you know that you've done some serious damage.

But often, injuries will sneak up on us. The reasons are many: bad form, an old injury that never healed right, pushing too hard for too long without adequate recovery, lack of adequate functional flexibility or joint stability, and of course pattern overload.

The trick with the first type of injury is pretty simple: don't be an idiot! If there is something obviously wrong, you need to let it heal.

Dealing with an Injury

The second type is trickier. How do you tell a growing injury from the soreness that will often accompany working out? The often recommended "see your doctor" is certainly never a bad idea, but unfortunately, short of some very expensive tests, your doctor really doesn't have any way of knowing the cause of your pain (x-rays will usually tell them nothing).

Their normal advice of over the counter pain medication, ice and rest may be safe advice from the physician's perspective, but is not always productive. Unless the pain is severe, common anti-inflammatory (NSAIDs) pain relievers, will not only mask the pain (possibly encouraging you to injure it further), but according to studies, may also slow the healing.[27,28,29]

Using NSAIDs, for common muscle soreness, will also slow the muscle building and recovery process as well, so it's a good idea to get out of the habit of using them unless really necessary for severe pain.

Icing the area is almost ALWAYS a good idea! There are various theories on the method of action of icing injuries, the most common being that it simply reduces inflammation, doesn't seem to really explain it. One theory that seems to make sense to me is that the transition from icing to not icing causes the body to flood the area with blood, which speeds the healing.

When icing an injury or possible injury, it is recommended that you get the area as cold as possible for 10-20 minutes, and then allow it to warm up. Repeat as often as possible.

Rest of course, is always needed for a real injury, but you won't make much progress if you take a week of rest every time you have some muscle soreness.

Just as with a defined injury, this is situation requires a little common sense: first, regardless of what you are doing (treadmill, squat rack, tennis), at the first sign of pain, stop what you are doing. Get off the treadmill, rack the weight, take a break, etc. Sometimes you just tweaked something and your body responded with a phantom pain, but it pays to stop, move the joint around a little, and see if the sensation is still there with no load.

I know my body well enough that I can pretty much tell right away when I need to back off for the day. At some point, hopefully you will as well. "Working through the pain" is never a good idea and will hurt you in the long run.

As long as the pain goes away when you stop doing what you were doing, you may be fine to move on to some other exercise. Be very careful that nothing else brings back the pain.

I've often noticed that pain that is very specific to one joint and occurs only when doing a specific movement, may be the result of bad form or joint angle, and sometimes, can be eliminated by simply altering hand or foot position. Your joints are not as simple or sturdy as the hinges on a door. They are held in place by muscles, tendons, and ligaments. It is very possible to force a joint into an angle that will lead to misalignment of the joint or pinching of tendons or ligaments.

For instance, I have found that how you hold and position your shoulders during upper body exercises can have a large affect on shoulder pain or injuries.

Another common alignment problem is allowing the knees to cave inward during squats, lunges, or even while doing cardio such as biking or stair climbing. A much of the knee pain most people experience can in fact be attributed to this one postural issue.

Back to what to do if you do experience pain while working out. If you do not experience any pain to the area when you are not working it, you should still take it easy on the area for a day or two. When you return to working it, go slow and light on the area at first, and stop immediately at any sign of discomfort. Work back up to your full intensity workout over several workouts.

If you feel any pain at all when NOT working that area of the body, you'll need to monitor it for the next couple of days. Ice the area, and be careful with any daily activities that may affect it. Even something as simple as sleeping on it wrong may aggravate a growing injury. If the area bothers you at all during normal activities, then odds are you have a soft tissue injury of some sort. Ice it as often as possible.

If you can come up with workouts that work around the injured area, you can still workout. I've worked out with broken legs, collarbones, etc. Where there's a will, there's a way. Do not try to work the affected area until the pain has completely subsided in normal activity, and any movement of the affected area brings on no discomfort. Ease back into it over the course of several workouts. If the pain comes back at any point, you probably have a chronic issue, and need to isolate the affected area even longer.

If you get to the point where you have been through the stop and go process several times, and have rested the area for longer than several weeks, and returning to working that area still causes the symptoms to return, it's time to see an orthopedic surgeon. Preferably, one who specializes in sports medicine. If they frequently work on athletes, they are more likely to take your goals seriously, and less likely to say something stupid like "just stop moving your arm above your head."

In my extensive experience, most significant reoccurring injuries suffered by your average fitness buff, started off as very minor ones. If they had been dealt with properly from the beginning, they would never have developed into anything major. Use your common sense!!

If you have an injury that isn't healing and you've already been to your doctor and they have been of little help, I am a big fan of a type of therapy called ART or Active Release Technique. ART is a quickly growing specialty that is very often practiced by sports therapists, but is available to normal people such as you and I. Go to my web site for a link to a practitioner in your area. If you have a reoccurring injury, you owe it to yourself to check out ART or one of the similar sports based therapeutic techniques.

There are other types of therapies as well. I would look for something very specific to sports injuries. I have found the physical therapy typically prescribed and paid for under most insurance plans to be inadequate for most of the injuries I see. Possibly not because of a lack of knowledge on the part of the therapists, as much as the fact that the time they have to work with you is so limited, and they are typically more interested in getting you back to functioning in normal life and are not particularly concerned with your goals in the gym.

Specific Injuries

There are more possible injuries than I could go into here. I'm going to spend a little space on the three I see most commonly. Much of what I go through with these can apply to other injuries as well.

Shoulder Injuries

The shoulder is a VERY complicated joint. In fact it's not so much a joint as a series of bones supported by muscles, tendons and ligaments. It's very easy to injure this joint and I'm not sure I know too many people who haven't injured one or both of their shoulders at some point.

Since there are so many ways to injure your shoulders, it would be impractical to try to delve deeply into all the injury modalities in this book, but I'll give you my most useful stretches and rehab/prehab "Complex." (see photos)

As I've mentioned elsewhere, current evidence indicates that static stretching before exercising can reduce strength in the stretched muscles. For some exercises, this may mean that you should wait until after working out to stretch, but for the shoulder, especially if you have shoulder issues, stretching before doing certain exercises may save you from possible issues. In this case, I recommend stretching after warming up and before any exercise that may force the shoulder into an "unnatural" range of motion. I'll even have some clients stretch their shoulders before doing squats, as reaching back to hold the bar is problematic for some.

The series of stretches I recommend consists of five different positions. The final two require that you rotate your hand to the rear, while the elbow moves forward.

The exercise "complex" is three related exercises that can be done one after the other on the same pulley setup. You'll need to lower the weight significantly after each exercise. Probably as much as 60% after the first exercise, and another 50% before the last exercise.

I've found that incorporating these stretches and this complex into a clients program will usually not only alleviate many shoulder issues, but also, if done before problems start to occur, will probably save you from having future issues.

Shoulder Stretches

Start the shoulder stretches with straight arm positions. You should feel a stretch in different parts of your shoulder and chest at each position. For the fourth and fifth positions the upper arm should point straight out from the shoulder. Rotate the forearm to the rear in the upper and lower position. You will need to use a vertical post such that your elbow can rest against the front while you grab the rear of the post with your hand. Rotate your body to get a gentle stretch. Hold for 10-20 seconds in each position. Repeat with the other arm.

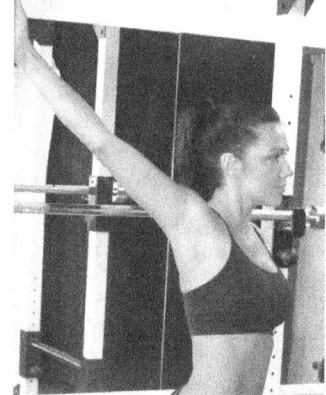

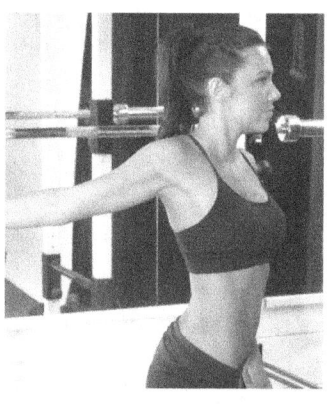

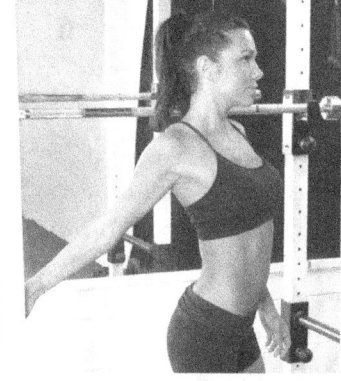

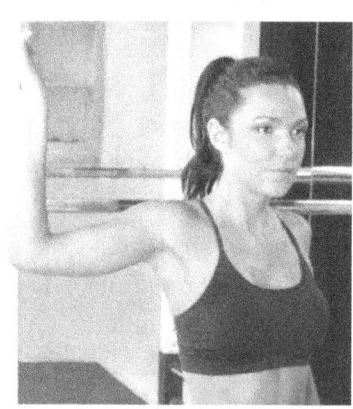

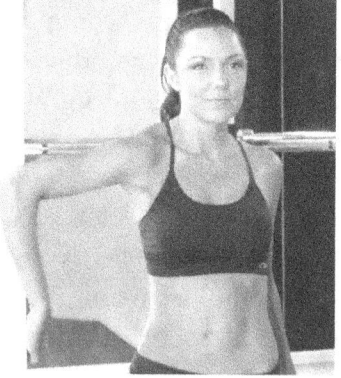

Shoulder Complex

These can be done with bands or a pulley machine. I prefer a good pulley. The first movement is a conventional one arm row. You will have to drop down almost 40% in weight for the second movement which is a high row to the side of the head. Notice the ending hand position with the palm rotated away. The palm should start facing the ground or slightly toward the body. The third movement will require a further drop in weight. Keep your upper arm straight out from the shoulder throughout. Rotate the forearm to the vertical position. Use a rep range of 10-12 for each. Repeat for the other arm.

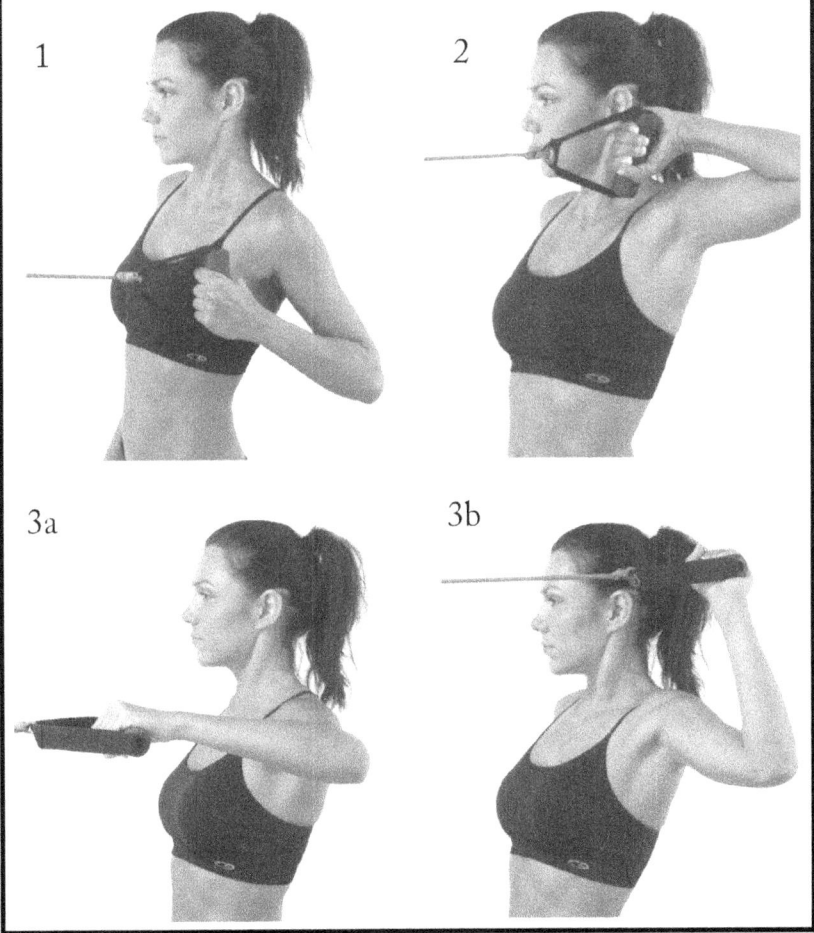

Lower Back Injuries

I've read that anywhere between 80% and 90% of us will experience back pain at some point in our lives. What makes this statistic even worse is that once the vast majority of people experience back pain for the first time, it never really goes away. Of even greater concern is that many causes of back pain remain unknown, and universally successful treatments have yet to be discovered.

If you have back pain that is severe and reoccurring, you should consider seeking medical attention for your condition. Get second and third opinions. Try various options including chiropractic and massage for muscle spasms. Surgery is being recommended less and less, and medicating with pain killers is usually only a temporary solution.

I'm writing this to advise you on the proper way to exercise in order to optimize back health. In fact, even if you have purely aesthetic goals, you'll also benefit from improved back health and core muscle strength resulting from a proper training plan as outlined here. This knowledge is from years of studying all the available research on the topic (I myself herniated a disk when I was younger, and only through proper exercise do I now have the strong and healthy back I do today), as well as working with perhaps hundreds of individuals who suffered from back pain before training with me. Indeed, one of my clients said after only two months of training: "I've had trouble getting out of bed every day for years because of my back, and I just noticed the other day that I haven't felt any pain in weeks. Do you think it has anything to do with our workouts?"

For optimal back health and strength, I'll outline some of the basics of proper training. First of all, it is important to be aware of the fact that your spine is supported by all the muscles in your midsection. To properly support your lower back throughout the course of normal day-to-day functions, the muscles of your lower back have to work in concert with your abs, oblique's, etc. Hence, I prefer to utilize exercises that transfer the load from the upper to lower body, or vice versa, in order to strengthen the core. I break these exercises down into two categories: 1) Heavy exercises that work on strengthening the core musculature with the spine in a straight (neutral) position, and 2) Light weight, high repetition exercises that work on muscular endurance and move the spine through a range of bending and twisting motions.

Heavy Exercises with a Static, Neutral Spine

Your spine is in a "neutral" position when you are standing straight with good posture. In this position, your back is actually capable of withstanding incredibly high loads without damage to your spine. When your back is in this position, you can work on strengthening the muscles of your lower back in a way that will improve your ability to lift heavy loads without injury. In fact, exercises like squats, deadlifts, rows, military presses, etc. will not only strengthen your lower back, but they will teach you to lift heavy objects with good form. These are compound, multi-joint exercises. Machines and single joint isolation exercises will NOT have the same benefits.

One VERY important note I know I spoke of this previously but it bears repeating: these exercises MUST be done with proper form or you will risk back injury. This means keeping the back flat during the entire range of motion. It's also important to brace your spine using your natural weight belt. This means you should tense the muscles around your waist similarly to the way a boxer braces for a punch to the stomach. Don't suck it in, just tense it.

The midsection of your body is analogous to a suspension bridge. Your spine is the main structure of the bridge, and the muscles are the guide wires. Without the guide wires the bridge would collapse under its own weight, but with properly loaded guide wires connecting and supporting each section of the bridge, it's able to support a heavy load. But like a bridge whose structure is dislodged by some sort of natural disaster, your back can only support heavy loads when the spine is aligned properly. Any bending or twisting of the spine throws this system off, and greatly reduces its load carrying capacity.

A study was done on weightlifters doing deadlifts to determine how they were able to repeatedly lift such monstrously heavy loads without any long-term back problems. The lifters performed repeated deadlifts while the positions of their spines were recorded in real time with specialized equipment. By chance, during one of the lifts, a lifter felt something go wrong and complained of lower back pain. Upon examining the video, it was found that for a brief moment during the lift, one of the lumbar joints went from a neutral to a flexed position for a brief instance. None of the other lifters complained of pain, and examination of all of their videos showed no other instances of their spines losing their neutral position. [30]

To summarize the last couple of paragraphs: If you're going to lift a heavy object, either in the gym, or in the real world, you MUST learn to bend at the hips so as to maintain a neutral spine position! If you learn one lesson from this chapter, this is probably the MOST important. I've found that perfecting the form on the Stiff Leg Deadlift is the best way to teach someone to lift properly. Once you mentally master this exercise, you will probably never hurt your lower back again!

Light Weight, High Rep

The other types of exercises that will help the lower back are muscular endurance exercises, which involve a range of bending and twisting (if your lower back is healthy). When you are bent over or twisting, your spine is in a very compromised position. If you try to lift a heavy load with your back rounded, the chances of getting a herniated disk are upwards of 100 times greater than with a flat back. In the real world, much of what we do involves bending and twisting. Hence, it is still necessary to strengthen the core musculature through these motions.

Since we don't want to put high loads on the spine in these compromised positions, we use lighter loads and higher repetitions to improve our muscular endurance. Since we shouldn't ever be lifting heavy loads in these positions, working on muscular endurance will go a long way towards taking the loads off the spine while you bend and twist in everyday movements. Some of the exercises I prefer for high rep work are swiss ball crunches, unloaded hyperextensions, front and side planks and various twisting exercises with cable machines or exercise tubing. These should be done with a load that you can do at least 15-20 reps.

Pull Throughs - With some of the newer multi-position cable machines you can do dozens of variations of this very practical exercise. High/low, one or two handed, etc.

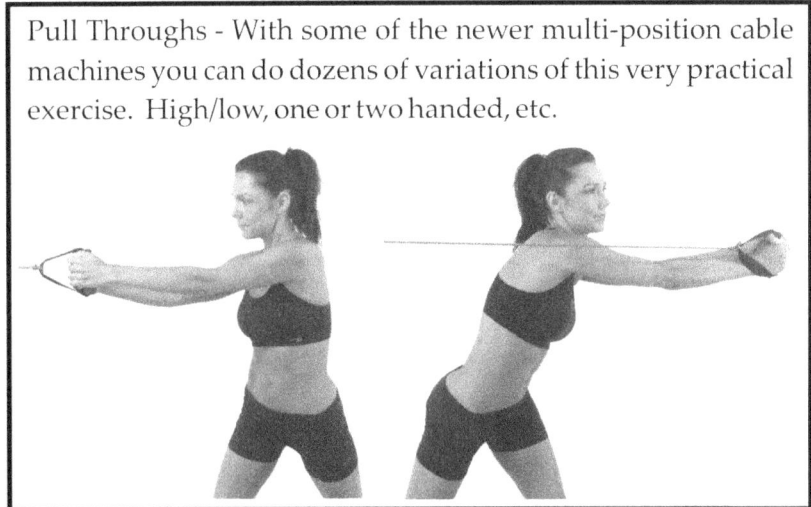

Back Rehab

For many years, common practice in the rehabilitation of a back injury was for the therapist to start you with the light weight, full range of motion exercises and progress to the more conventional lifts. However, it is best to limit the range of motion of the spine until injuries are fully healed. Remember, flexing will almost always be detrimental to a damaged spine. In fact, I've had clients who couldn't do a single crunch without waking up in pain the next morning, and yet could do proper, stiff leg deadlifts without pain.

If you have been treated for a back injury, and your doctor has cleared you to start exercising again, the following is my preferred progression:

1. Start with a general-purpose, full body routine. All exercises should use light weight to start, and meticulous attention should be paid to making sure the spine stays in a neutral position throughout. The only core exercises that should be performed at this point are static planks (front and side). A front plank is similar to a push-up off your elbows and toes, except that you just hold the position. Side planks are the same, except facing to the side.

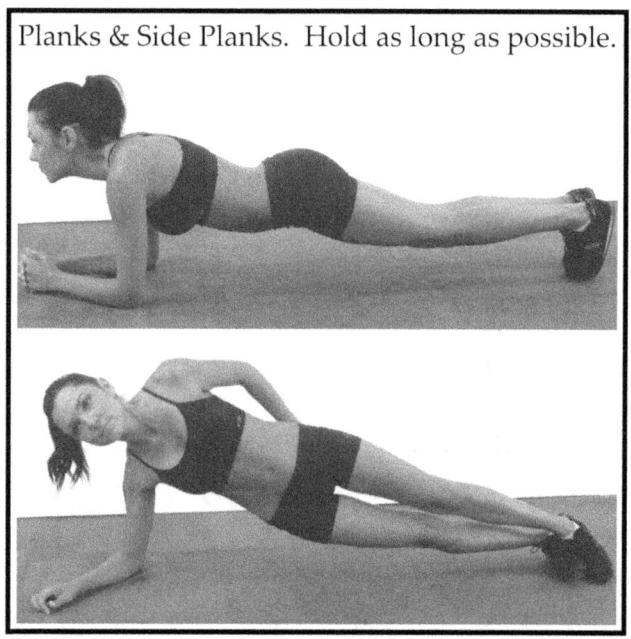

Planks & Side Planks. Hold as long as possible.

For cardio, do plenty of fast walking. Studies have shown walking fast (at a pace where the arms swing), is distinctly better for a recovering back than slow walking or running.[31] Stop ANY exercise if pain is experienced. This is not a toughman competition, and pain is a warning sign that should not be ignored!

2. Build up the weight gradually. Realize you will have good days and bad days. Don't force yourself to go heavier with each workout if you don't feel up for it. Do not let anyone persuade you into doing balance or stability exercises at this point (exercises that require sitting or standing on an unsteady surface), as this is an easy way to accidentally put the spine into a compromised position where it could be reinjured.

3. Once you have gone a month or so without any pain and your weights are back to normal, you can slowly reintegrate bending and twisting exercises. Start with small range of motion crunches on a padded floor, and work up from there. Again, if a particular exercise causes pain, stop immediately and go back a step.

4. Don't be discouraged if it takes a long time to return to normal. Depending on the actual cause of the pain, certain parts of your back may take a long time to heal, even under the best conditions. Some injuries are severe enough that they will NEVER heal completely. If you truly herniated a disk, chances are you will have to deal with it for the rest of your life. At that point bending and twisting will always be problematic, and should be minimized. From then on, you'll really have to concentrate on using your hips and legs not your lower back.

In the past, conventional wisdom was to stretch the back to help restore range of motion. This may feel good in the short term, but recent studies have shown any stretching of an injured back will cause more damage. Range of motion in the spine is actually not very important to overall back health.[32]

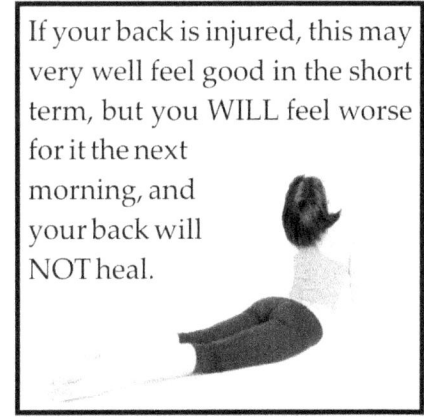

If your back is injured, this may very well feel good in the short term, but you WILL feel worse for it the next morning, and your back will NOT heal.

Another warning is in regards to bed rest. Although it might be recommended in some extreme cases, most studies have shown bed rest slows the healing process.[33] Get up, move around, take a walk, and get back into life. Just be careful of your activities until the pain subsides.

Remember, I'm not a doctor. This information is based on the latest research in conjunction with my own personal experiences. Individual results may vary, and you should always consult your physician whenever in doubt. [iii,iv]

Knee Injuries

The knee is a rather simple joint as human joints go, but since it is so highly loaded and so often abused, injuries are common.

Unfortunately, as with much in health and fitness, the "authorities" are usually pushing people in the absolutely incorrect direction. "Squats are bad for the knees" and other such nonsense keeps many people from having the strong leg muscles that will actually prevent knee injuries, and the advice most physicians will give: "don't ever do squats again" will keep many people from ever recovering fully from knee injuries.

Many times, patients with damaged cartilage will even be told to avoid walking due to the "impact." Unfortunately, keeping the joint strong and controlled is the only way to maintain joint integrity. If you are not walking and keeping the joint strong, ANY motion will result in improper "meshing" of the cartilage interface and result in damage. It has even been theorized that impact and loading will slowly result in cartilage regenerating (still speculative), which would make sense as that is how the rest of the body works.

While there are certainly some injuries where healing time is necessary and some circumstances where severe injuries will totally preclude loaded bending of the knee joint, this is actually rare.

Remember, it's the muscles that support the joint and enable the bones to ride correctly on the cartilage. The stronger the

182

muscles are, the better controlled the motion will be. Your body was BUILT to walk and squat down fully, and it's only in our culture that full squatting isn't a normal part of everyday life. When a strongly supported knee moves through these motions, even slightly damaged cartilage will prevent any further damage. If the muscles of the knee are not kept strong, then any motion of the knee will cause damage.

Other than traumatic injury and damage caused by weak supporting musculature, probably the most common cause of knee injuries is bad form while squatting or jumping. Particularly allowing the knees to bow inward. As discussed earlier, this is particularly common among women due to the structural differences of the hips, but is not rare in men either. In a high percentage of the individuals who tell me they have knee pain during squatting, I will see this inward bowing.

One of the best ways I have found to cure this habit is to tie an elastic band, around the knees pulling inward. While this may seem counterproductive, the unnatural force of the band pulling inward will force you to consciously push outward to resist. A couple of months of this and you will learn good form that hopefully will last.

A great deal of attention is usually paid to the advice of not allowing the knees to go past the toes during squats, lunges, or similar exercises. However, studies have shown that although the shearing force on the knee does increase somewhat the further forward the knee goes, it is not generally considered significant enough to worry about. Making an effort to keep the knees behind the toes will result in much greater stress on the lower back.[34] Your personal limb lengths will determine where your knees end up. As long as you are using good form overall, you shouldn't have issues.

Allowing the knees to bow inward during squatting and especially during jumping and landing is common and very destructive. A good coach should look out for this especially in female athletes in jumping sports. In the gym you can cure this bad habit with some elastic exercise tubing around the knees while squatting.

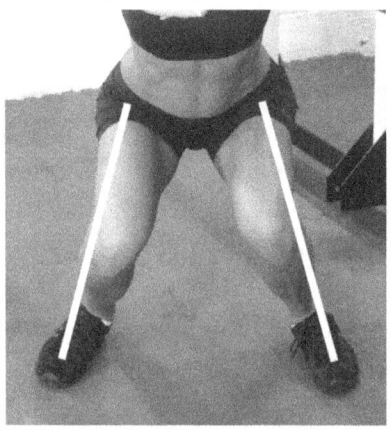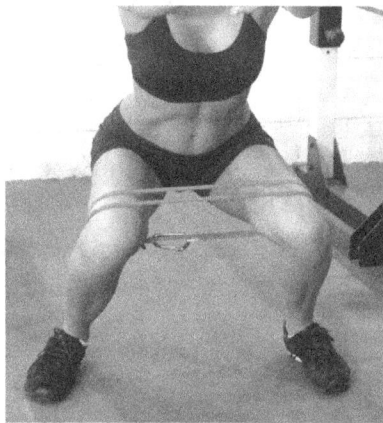

A lot of discourse is also put into the depth you should use when squatting and doing similar exercises. While many feel a shallow squat is less damaging, I feel that the evidence supports the fact that you really do need to strengthen this joint through a full range of motion. The knee joint is actually stronger when bent past 90 degrees than it is at the critical angle where many will choose to change direction.

Besides, most fans of using a partial range of motion in squatting movements are really only using this bad logic to support their own egos. Let's face it, full range of motion squats are SERIOUSLY HARD WORK, and most tough guys would have to take way too much weight off the bar in order to do them correctly. Full range squats will never really damage their knees, but in order to do them correctly, their egos would be seriously bruised.

Don't forget deadlifts and leg curls either. To prevent injuries, a strong knee needs to be supported by the muscles on both sides of the legs.

Leg extensions tend to take a pretty serious beating in the exercise science scene, and for good reason. It is a very unnatural load on the knee joint, and places shear stress on this joint that is many times higher than in a properly done squat. I will never go so far as to say you should avoid this exercise completely, but try not to use them continually, and certainly abstain from leg extensions if you are having knee pain issues!

This is just a partial list of the injuries you may have to deal with, however much of the advice will apply to other joints as well. Of course, my hope is that you will never need to apply the information in this section.

Chapter 12 - Misc. Exercise Topics

Posture

One huge factor in the appearance and function of your body is posture. I am continually amazed at just how underrated posture is with the general public. It's not underrated in fashion, sports, dance, or many other activities, but the general public seems to wander around oblivious to the fact that the way they hold themselves has such a great effect on how they look and feel.

In fact, most people do know good posture when they see it, they just can't indentify that's what they are seeing, nor do they realize when their own posture is bad. On many occasions, I've heard friends say things like "That guy walks around like he owns the place" or "She really grabs my attention, but I don't know why." That's when I give them the answer: it's because they have great posture!

Great posture will make you look more confident, taller and thinner. It will give guys the look of a stronger, broader chest, and will give girls not only an apparent cup size increase, but will give you a "lift" that even the best bra can't duplicate, as well as eliminating that "pooch" some women are always complaining about.

Why do I bring up posture in a health and fitness book? Because although you can force yourself to have good posture to some extent, if you want really good posture all the time, even without thinking about it, the only way you're going to get and keep it is through a properly balanced resistance training program. The words "properly balanced" are critical here. Even most fitness buffs usually have routines that do not result in an overall balanced musculature.

I see two prevalent postural errors in the majority of the clients I work with. There are other small areas of bad posture, but these two are so wide spread, so prevalent, and so blatant that by taking care of these two, you'll be 90% of the way there. In fact, I've found that if you take care of these two, a couple others will go away as well.

Forward Pelvic Tilt

By far the postural error most complained about among women is forward pelvic tilt. If you look at someone from the side, with a properly adjusted belt, the belt should be nearly level to the ground. In almost all of you, your belt will be much lower at the front than at the back.

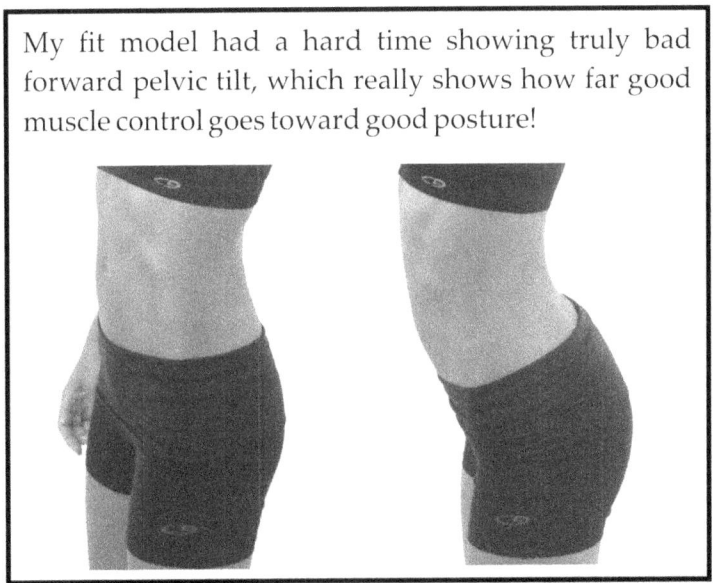

My fit model had a hard time showing truly bad forward pelvic tilt, which really shows how far good muscle control goes toward good posture!

This has a couple of negative effects visually. First, it affects the posture of the rest of your upper body. Since you are now angled forward at the waist, you will be compensating all the way up through your neck. Especially for women, this will result in what many of you call your "pooch", or the little belly that sticks out even if you're not over weight. Many will attribute this to child birth or getting older, but it's really not a function of your belly at all. If you correct the forward pelvic tilt, the "pooch" will go away. The forward pelvic tilt will also make you look shorter, as it creates an "S" curve through your upper body. You will never stand straight, and you'll look it.

What causes this? Beyond intentional bad posture caused by lack of self-esteem or tall girl syndrome, it's pretty straight forward: tight quads and hip flexors along with weak lower posterior chain musculature (glutes, hamstrings). The reason this postural imbalance is so prevalent is because these two weaknesses are so common. I won't speculate as to why most people have tight quads and hip flexors, other than the fact that we don't do nearly enough activities with our lower bodies that use a truly full range of motion. We're all tight there.

I'm not going to get into the details of flexibility and stretching in this book, as if I did, this would quickly turn into a 500 page book, but there are no end of free internet resources that will tell you how to stretch your quads, and hip flexors. Check out my web site for some good ones.

The reason for the weak lower posterior chain muscles was discussed earlier: we just don't use them in our modern lifestyles. Both the glutes and hamstrings get utilized when we pick up heavy objects with PROPER form (something no one does), bending at the hips, keeping the back flat, and using these muscles instead of the lower back. I do not know why the muscles of the lower back are the "lazy" way of picking things up, but they are.

For week glutes and hams, the number one best exercise BY FAR is the stiff leg dead lift described earlier.

This one exercise alone will do more for your physical appearance than perhaps any other exercise. I'm not saying this is the be-all, end-all of exercises, but if you're not doing this exercise, you're really missing out.

The other activity that will really help is sprinting. Jogging and running will not work the glutes, or hams to any significant extent. Only during true sprinting will these muscles become active. In the cardio chapter we talked about intervals. Intervals are more than just sprinting, but sprinting is certainly one of the most productive ways to do intervals.

There are reasons Olympic sprinters have such enviably toned physiques, and it's not because of long slow cardio, or even endless hours in the gym. Sprinting itself may be one of the most productive ways of exercising. The muscular and cardio benefits are many.

Even if you do have a healthy heart, you still need to worry about pulling a muscle, rolling an ankle, or otherwise hurting yourself. You'd think sprinting would be such a natural activity, but you don't realize how unnatural it is until you try it (for the first time perhaps in decades)! If you do feel like you are up to it, start out slowly. Run fast for a couple intervals. Work up to sprinting over the course of many workouts.

What separates sprinting from running? When you sprint, not only does neither foot touch the ground at the same time (unlike jogging), but your heels also never touch the ground. When you're sprinting you pretty much float from the toes and balls of one foot to the other foot.

It really is that foreign of an activity. As strange as it seems, you just don't ever sprint, even when you think you're running really fast. It's an activity that has been removed from modern society, but one that uses certain muscles that just don't get used in other activities.

Yes, I'm a big fan of sprinting and stiff leg deadlifts! It's also not a bad thing that these exercises will really firm up your rear. No, there is no such thing as spot reduction, but since most people have almost no appreciable muscle in this area, once they lose the extra weight, their rear is still flabby. As you strengthen this area, you'll notice the droopy line that separates your butt from your upper legs will start to disappear, and any cellulite will greatly diminish (or disappear entirely) as the muscle that the skin is connected to starts to take on the size and shape it had when you were younger.

As an added benefit of making this postural improvement, you will start to use better form when you bend to pick things up. Your lower back will REALLY thank you.

Slumped Shoulders

The second postural imbalance most everyone has is shoulders that slump forward. From the standpoint of overall posture, this appears to be just a continuance of the forward pelvic tilt. From the side, your body forms an "S" shape. There is a correlation between the forward pelvic tilt and the slumped shoulders and just as there are various degrees of pelvic tilt, there is a huge range of slumped shoulders from really good to terrible. Most people fall into the middle zone where it's not overly apparent to others, but when corrected, makes a huge difference in appearance. Some, however, are so bad it becomes obvious.

Again, ignoring the possible intentional reasons for a slumped posture, how do you correct it? This one is very simple. Although tight pecs are part of the problem, the majority of the solution is in one exercise: rows. High row, low rows, dumbbell, barbell, pulley, etc. etc. For the upper body, rows are probably the number one neglected exercise, hence the slumping shoulders.

Guys neglect rows because they spend too much time benching. Girls neglect rows because they have never been taught otherwise, or they think pressing will help expand their chest. In both cases, we can see our chest, but the back is neglected because we don't look at it in the mirror. As straightforward as this may seem, unfortunately both sexes have it backwards. Not only will working the chest more than the back (doing more presses than rows), screw up your posture, it will also not give you the results you are looking for.

The slumped shoulders on the left is NOT an exaggeration. I see worse all the time, but it was as bad as my model could imitate.

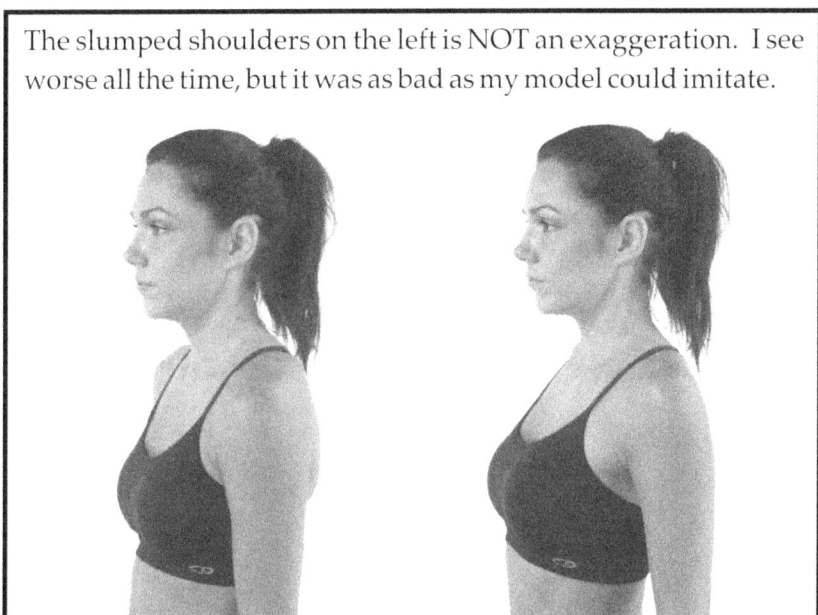

Yes, bench pressing is the exercise that will work the chest most effectively, however the pectoral muscles of the chest are actually pretty small in comparison to the various back muscles. For a guy, working the back muscles will actually make you look thicker and more muscular than will working the chest. Couple that with the fact that the improved posture (shoulders pulled back) will actually make the chest look much bigger.

This is true for women as well. I'm not saying every woman is looking for bigger breasts, but it's pretty standard for women to appear at least one cup size bigger with the correct "shoulder back" posture. Even if you have no desire to look a cup size bigger, having the correct posture will make them stand higher and give your body a younger look, as well as helping to eliminate the lower back pain many well-endowed women complain of.

This section was by no means meant to be a complete resource on posture. As with the rest of this book, it's just meant to cover the issues I've seen most often. If appearance is one of your goals, do NOT overlook this topic!

Core (Abs)

The science behind a six pack (or at least the perceived science), has changed a number of times over the years. Hence, so have my thoughts on how we should work our abs. However, one thing has not changed: no matter how many people I have worked with, I have never seen anyone go from pot belly to ripped six pack by doing endless crunches, sit-ups, pilates or any other exercise.

First we have to take a step back and examine why we have this obsession with dedicated ab exercises such as sit-ups and crunches. Of course everyone wants a flat stomach, and some of you would REALLY like to have a "six-pack" as well. The problem is, sit-ups have little to do with a flat stomach. In fact, we all have a six-pack. It's just that most of us have buried it under a layer of fat. Remove the fat, and we all have beautiful abs.

Most of you should know by now that there's no such thing as "spot reduction." Your body takes fat from all areas of your body. It doesn't care what area you're working. Working the abs will in no way make the fat disappear from around your midsection. In fact, if fat loss is your goal, then spending endless hours doing crunches is a terrible way to go. Your abs are very small in comparison to your legs and all the other muscles in your body. Why not work the muscles that really burn calories? Remember, we're trying for the most efficient workout

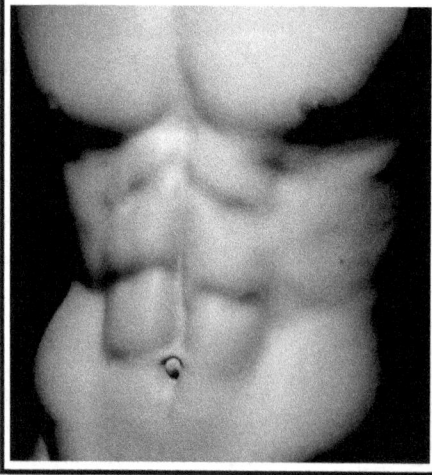

Unfortunately, a six-pack is more a function of a lack of body fat covering the muscles than how many crunches you do.

possible here. Just going through an inefficient program because it makes us feel good about our workout, is not what we're after.

Ab work is definitely one of those topics where we have to go back to the introduction and remember that everyone is different, and more importantly, everyone has different goals, and different limitations. My recommendations are very different for a competitive boxer and a female model, and although a strong midsection is important to both a healthy high school football player and 45-year-old executive who has struggled with bad back pain at various points of his life the methods will be different.

I am not entirely convinced that this is a big factor for many people, but from what I've seen, too much direct ab work will in fact give some people a thick mid-section. This isn't a big factor for guys or for anyone that still has some body fat to lose, but if you're a trim female looking for that hourglass figure, too much core work is counterproductive (i.e. Pilates). As an example of this, go back and checkout a photo of Britney Spears when she first came onto the pop scene. Then compare it to a photo of the pop diva sometime around 2003-2004 after she dedicated herself to being as fit as possible. You'll notice that although she definitely looks super fit, the tinny trim waist she had a few years earlier was distinctly thicker. I can't tell you a thing about Britney's workouts back in those days, but I'm going to guess it includes several hundred crunches (or something comparable) everyday.

I wouldn't recommend getting too paranoid about this. I don't think anyone is going to get a thick midsection from doing the proper amount of core work, but it is possible to overdo it. Just as with every other aspect of fitness I talk about, you need to be aware of your goals, and how your program is going to get you there.

Of course there are more reasons than a six-pack to work our abs. Whether you want to be a Strongman, or just want to be functional and free of back-pain, having a strong mid-section is essential. Having a strong mid-section also helps for posture (looking good). A boxer or MMA athlete has to have an incredibly strong midsection that stays in an almost constant state of tension in order to protect the mid section from repeated punches, and without the athlete having to think about protecting himself.

For this athlete, there probably isn't a "too much ab work". But, for the person who has had back pain issues (80% of us at some point in our lives), we need to be very careful of overdoing it. Especially with ab work that requires any sort of bending and twisting.

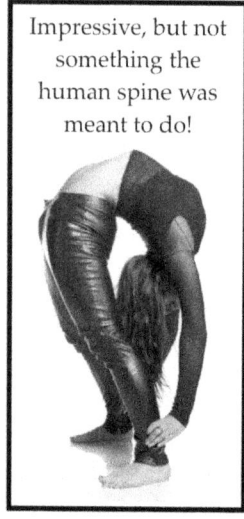

Impressive, but not something the human spine was meant to do!

The unfortunate fact of life is that once you've damaged your spine through misuse or simply by allowing yourself to get so out of shape that you develop back issues through otherwise normal daily activities, it will probably never heal completely. You may be able to stay pain free with proper workouts, however, trying to emulate the workouts of the above mentioned boxer, will probably bring the pain back.

As we discussed earlier, the current line of thinking is that our core is not built so much for moving our upper body in relation to our lower body, but to stabilize it. That's right, flexing through the spine may be a bad idea regardless of how strong your core is. Take female gymnasts for example. Watch how far they can contort their bodies, arching their backs so far they can touch their feet to the backs of their heads. Unfortunately, competitive gymnasts also have incredibly high incidences of lower back disorders later in life. These repeated contortions destroy their spines regardless of how strong their core is.

Unfortunately, the take home message here is not well defined. For some, working their core through a full range of motion is almost required, and not particularly harmful, whereas to others, ab work should only be of the type designed to stabilize the core, not move it. Only a thorough knowledge of your own body will enable you to determine where you stand.

We also have to remember that the rectus abdominis (the six pack) rarely acts alone in contraction. In fact it almost always acts in conjunction with many other muscles including the external and internal obliques, transversus abdominis, latimus dorsi, erector spinae, psoas minor and major, iliacus, and more. These muscles act as a natural weight belt to stabilize the spine and hold or move the midsection. Paying too much attention to the rectus abdominis isn't going to strengthen your midsection unless you're also strengthening all those other muscles.

For a while, weighted ab exercise was in style. The theory was that high rep work did very little to actually strengthen the core muscles. Many of the current experts on back health are starting to turn back the clock to the days of higher rep ab work. Unlike other muscles in the body, your core muscles need to be activated to some degree all of the time. In fact, you should probably try to concentrate on contracting your core muscles a little bit even while you are seated. A slouched and relaxed posture while sitting can be one of the big factors in developing lower back issues.

It seems the jury is still out on this issue, but I think the consensus is that you should look to keep the rep range for core work in the 15-30 rep range. I'm sure I will change my opinion on that at some point, but the message here is that doing weighted crunches in the 5-10 rep range or doing 200 sit-ups, are both probably not productive.

Working Your Abs

So how should we be training our abs? Yes, we may do some swiss ball crunches, just as we may do some curls for the biceps, but mainly we're training the core with planks, unilateral exercises (one limb at a time), squats, deadlifts, presses, rows, pull-downs, and full body cable twists. We're doing full body movements that use our abs as they were meant to be used: to stabilize the upper and lower halves of the body. If you're not doing full body exercises, you'll need a lot more dedicated core work.

I am particularly fond of planks, full body cable pulls and one arm pressing movements. Planks are great for teaching yourself to actively "connect" the upper and lower halves of your body. A plank looks just like a push-up at the top position, except that you are resting on your toes, elbows and forearms not your toes and hands. You hold that position for as long as you can. It helps to time it and keep trying to go longer. Once you reach two minutes, you may want to try putting a small weight on your back to make the exercise harder.

You will also want to try these on your side as well to work the obliques and other core muscles. I will usually start in the standard position and rotate to the sides as I get tired. I'll keep rotating back and forth between the three positions as long as I can. See the photos in the section on back health.

One arm pressing movements are pretty simple. Whether it's a bench press or military press, if you are using enough weight, you should really feel it in your core, as you transfer the weight from the active arm through your core to the legs which are either holding you up or stabilizing you side to side.

Full body cable pulls are great exercises in general. I love how they work almost the entire body in a very functional manner. Form is very important on these, as you should really be twisting through the legs, hips shoulders and arms, not through the lower back. In fact, part of the exercise is concentrating on contracting the core so as to not allow rotation through the lower back at or at least minimize it. Again, see the photos in the section on back health.

One caveat here!!!! Since most of you have never really trained the core in a functional way, most of you will start out very imbalanced. Combine that with a typical beginner's bad form, and it becomes easy to injure your back. Not that the muscles in your back won't occasionally be sore (just like the other muscles you worked), but you have been ignoring those muscles for years, and they have a lot of catching up to do.

This isn't to say we're never going to work the rectus abdominis with a couple sets of stability ball crunches, but not to the extent some people do. Don't use the "I don't want blocky abs" excuse I just gave you to avoid ab work altogether.

As far as that six-pack is concerned, just keep up those workouts, keep the diet clean, and you too can have a beautiful midsection without hours of crunches. For those of you that hate crunches, don't get too happy....we'll find many more exercises you'll hate even more.

Stretching

I'm not going to spend a lot of time on stretching because there is so much conflicting information out there on this topic, that my mind is not totally made up on the How, When and How Much of stretching. There are many books out there on stretching (check out my web site), and lacking any conclusive studies either way, I really can't vouch for any one method over another.

Therein lies the big issue: everyone seems to have their own opinion on stretching, how much is necessary, how to do it, etc. A couple of years ago, a study came out saying that stretching didn't reduce injuries in athletes. A lot of people were up in arms about the study, and although the conclusion was a bit broad given the scope of the study, the point is well taken: many of our preconceived notions about stretching may not be true.

One change in popular opinion that seems to be catching on is that stretching a muscle before working it can reduce the weight you can lift and therefore the effectiveness of the workout. However sometimes, stretching the antagonist (the muscle that would normally oppose the motion), may help you lift more. That may be more complicated than you need to get but it's a good example of how sketchy our knowledge of stretching really is.

I've also found that many individuals have tight muscles in areas that will restrict the motion of the exercise and that stretching pre-exercise will help the workout, even though that muscle is involved in the motion. A good example is that I've found a majority of beginning lifters are restricted in the range of motion they can get in the squat by tight calf muscles. Hence stretching the soleus (the section of the calf muscle that is activated when the knee is bent), is a standard part of my pre squat routine for most people.

How much should you stretch? It depends how much stretching you need. I know, kind of a lame answer, but without working with you directly there's really no good answer. I feel strongly that there is such a thing as too much stretching for many people, and although tight muscles and connective tissue may be restricting the range of motion of a particular joint, it is very possible to stretch that connective tissue to a point where it no longer properly supports the joint. At some point, the structure of the joint itself actually gets in the way and then you are doing more harm than good.

You may say "But people who do yoga all the time are way more flexible than I am. I've obviously got a long way to go before I've stretched too much." The problem is we're not all meant to be yoga instructors.

There is no doubt that some people are hypermobile (joints are constructed for a large range of motion) and some are hypomobile (small range of motion). This is biological fact. Some people will never be super flexible no matter how much they try, and continued effort to stretch the joints too far will result in weakening the connective tissue.

Yes, in effect, what I am saying is that for the most part, yoga masters were born, not made. I am of the opinion that this is why some people find yoga so satisfying and others can't stand it. If you're just not a flexible person, even the most common moves will always prove frustrating.

I am in no way saying anything bad about yoga. If you enjoy it, then great, it's a great addition to a well rounded fitness program.

I do warn against some of the recent attempts at turning yoga into something it isn't. "Power Yoga" is no more of a well rounded fitness program than those silly cardio classes that give you pink five pound dumbbells and try to persuade you that you're getting some sort of resistance training. Use yoga for what it's intended for: stretching and stress relief.

Tips For Stretching:

- Be careful of injuring your lower back!!! This point is huge! If you have ANY lower back issues at all, you should not be attempting to stretch your back out at all. Back injuries never fully heal and although stretching out the lower back might make it feel better in the short term, you will aggravate the injury long term.[35] This is important with traditional stretching as well as yoga. There are many yoga moves that someone with a lower back injury should simply not attempt. Many leg stretches, particularly anything for the glutes or

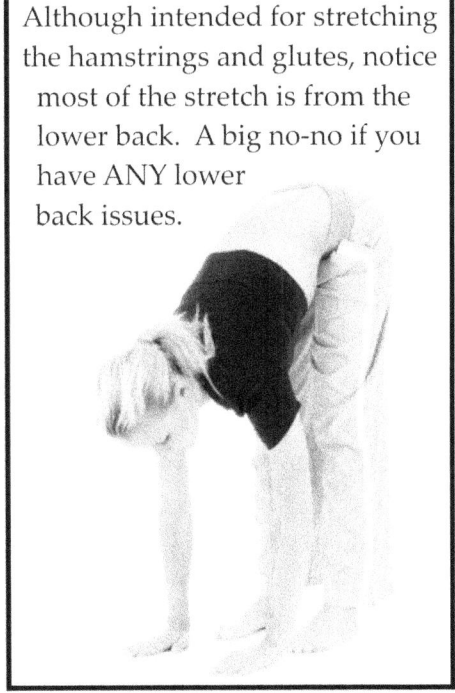

Although intended for stretching the hamstrings and glutes, notice most of the stretch is from the lower back. A big no-no if you have ANY lower back issues.

hamstrings, require careful attention to form. It is very easy to bend with the lower back while trying to do these stretches.

- Be strategic with your stretching. Only stretch muscles that need stretching before your workout. Learning what your body needs is a huge part of the workout puzzle. I can't tell you what stretches you'll find beneficial at what point in your workout, but I know what my body needs, and you need to figure out what yours needs.

- A good time for stretching is after your workout while your muscles are warm, but I prefer during my workout. By doing one specific stretch between two exercises, it gives me a short rest break during the workout, and allows me to utilize the time more efficiently. DO schedule some time for stretching. If you don't put it in your plan, you'll probably forget to do it at all.

- If you are particularly flexible in one area, there may be no real need for stretching that area. Concentrate on the muscles that are tight or restricting your motion

- Be careful with dynamic or ballistic stretching. Many trainers are a fan of this style of stretching, where you move quickly through the movements, bouncing at the end of the stretch. However, most experts feel this is a good way to injure yourself, and since it triggers the stretch reflex, and doesn't allow the muscle to relax at the end of the movement, it may very well defeat the purpose of the stretch.[36]

Ok, there you have it, a short section on stretching. Maybe by the time we get to the second edition there will be some more conclusive evidence to report. For now, just remember that moderation is key. A stretching program that is too aggressive may very well be almost as bad for you as not enough.

Exercise for Children and Teens

This is a topic that is very personal for me. I was overweight and out of shape as a child. The fact that I was overweight as a child has made it exponentially harder to stay in shape as an adult. I've read more research on this than I would want to get into, but the best evidence for me has been my clients. Beyond any doubt, I can always tell how difficult it will be for someone to get back into shape by how fit and athletic they were as a child.

I look around and see what is justifiably an epidemic of overweight children walking around and it really makes me sad. Most of them will never overcome this handicap, and will suffer serious, often deadly effects from this condition. Those who do overcome it later in life will always struggle because of it. Over 33% of all children ages 6-19 are currently overweight or obese. This figure has tripled since 1980.[37] Overweight adolescents have a 70 percent chance of becoming overweight or obese adults, and I think we all know the health risks involved in being an overweight adult.

Nearly one third of all US children eat fast food on a daily basis, and it continually amazes me the excuses parents make for feeding their vulnerable children this poison.

This is a major problem, not only for these children, but also for society, as health care costs continue to skyrocket, obesity related illness is a major factor. Seeing the trend start so early in life does not bode well for the future health of America. This next generation could conceivably be the first in recorded history to have an average lifespan less than their parents!

Ok, so enough with the scare tactics. If you don't already take the fitness of your children seriously, there's probably nothing I can do here to persuade you otherwise, but hopefully the fact that you've made it this far in the book says that you do indeed take it seriously.

What can you do about it? First of all, stop feeding them crap. Follow the same recommendations I make in the nutrition section for the entire family. Sorry if this sounds harsh, but making the excuse "my kids won't eat that healthy stuff" sounds pretty lame when you think about the fact that YOU ARE THEIR PARENTS!

Another excuse I hear from parents is "I don't want to turn my kids into anorexics." While it is true that anorexia is a serious issue, it pales in comparison to obesity. Your children are more than 10 times as likely to suffer serious health consequences from obesity as from anorexia. Good studies are hard to find, but as a direct comparison, in Canada (usually similar to the US) in 2004, 71 people between the age of 12 and 44 died from eating disorders like anorexia nervosa and bulimia nervosa. On the opposite side of the scale, there were 10,271 deaths due to obesity related disease in people from 12 to 44 years old that same year.

One fact almost all experts agree with: teaching your children proper eating habits and enforcing those habits will NOT lead to anorexia, but WILL help prevent obesity! Your own habits will probably do more good than anything. As with most of parenting, setting a good example is the best way to teach good habits. Think of that the next time you think "I'm too busy being a parent to exercise."

Exercise

This leads us to exercise. All the good eating habits in the world won't do much good if your children spend their day in front of the TV or computer. Many experts are saying that it is more the lack of exercise than bad nutrition causing the current explosion of childhood obesity.

I don't think we need a lot of statistics to know that the current generation spends a lot less time entertaining themselves in active ways than did past generations. If you are over 40, I'm sure you remember being sent out of the house at dawn, and not returning till dinner, all the while running, biking, playing your own version of baseball or other activity.

It simply amazes me how seldom I see children out playing in my very family oriented neighborhood. How do we fix this? Unfortunately, times have changed, and while past generations allowed children to play unsupervised, modern society judges the world to no longer be safe enough for this. So now children must join leagues and teams in order to be active. Parents are then required to sit on their butts on bleachers any and every time their children are doing anything active. Besides simply incorporating yourself in your children's sports and activities, I have little in the way of advice, but I can make some recommendations and dispel some myths.

Sports are probably the number one way for children to stay in shape. Sports add greatly to a child's development, mentally and physically, as well as socially. I highly recommend encouraging your children to play a variety of sports and activities. Even if you have dreams of seeing your son playing in the Super Bowl, letting him be a one sport athlete before he reaches a college level will not help his chances in the NFL but may hamper the development of his overall athletic ability and perhaps set him up for overuse injuries.

Female Athletes

At the risk of sounding sexist, I'm going to give some advice that really is based on sound biological fact. Young female athletes really are different from young male athletes. Men and women are constructed different in general, but the consequences of not taking this into account are more pronounced in youth.

The structure of the female hips is more compromised by the ability to have children than is the male body. The increased angle the legs take away from the hips makes it very easy for a young female athlete to have knee issues due to improper form when jumping, landing, running and cutting. Young female athletes are over 3 times as likely to suffer ACL injuries as male athletes.[38] Watch your female athlete on the court. When she jumps, do her knees stay in line with her hips and feet, or do they rotate in towards each other? Videotaping her playing will help you see this. Look at the photo in the section on knee injuries to see what it looks like when the knees rotate in.

You can help your young female athlete out in two ways. First, get them proper instruction from a good strength coach. They should spend time in the weight room doing quality lower body exercises to strengthen all the muscles around the knees. Teaching them proper form will help tremendously. Make sure the couch uses methods similar to what you see in this book. Machines are a big no-no for what we're looking to accomplish here because we're specifically looking to strengthen stabilizers and teach proper form and motion of the lower body, which will never happen with machines.

The other thing you can do is encourage her to play sports that emphasize form. This will certainly come off as sexist, no matter how I say it, but the fact remains, there is a distinct reason dance and gymnastics have long been a staple for athletic young women: they really do emphasize form such that your young female athlete will learn how to move properly.

Just as I've observed that adults who played sports as children get back in shape much quicker as adults than those who didn't, I know immediately when an adult female has been a dancer or gymnast. Their posture and coordination really do tend to be far better than other women, even those who played other sports.

Children and the Gym

What if your child wants to come to the gym with you? Don't' worry about all the old wives tales you've heard. There's nothing wrong with children of any age participating in gym based workouts as long as they follow some recommendations.

Almost all experts agree. The number one danger to children in the gym is lack of proper supervision. Properly supervised, the gym is a very safe environment for children. Left on their own, they will very easily find a way to hurt themselves. This also leads into proper training. Children should be educated in proper form for all exercises before they are allowed to lift heavier weights.

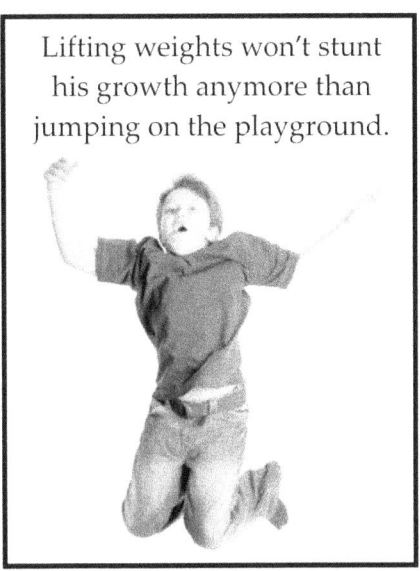

Lifting weights won't stunt his growth anymore than jumping on the playground.

The myth that children shouldn't lift weights because it will stunt their growth is simply not true. In fact several studies have completely disproven it. A child's bones and joints are stressed more jumping around on the playground than they ever are in the gym.[39,40,41,42]

Children can quickly make neuromuscular gains that will not only improve physical strength but may also improve muscular coordination. Recent studies are also showing that it may even be possible for children to put on healthy amounts of lean muscle through resistance training. This will aid the child not only in body composition, and sports performance, but also in injury prevention.[43]

Although very high volume training may not be the best for young children (Marathon training, etc.), moderate amounts of any type of aerobic activity are very healthy for children of all ages.

None of this will have long-term success unless the child enjoys the activity. Parents and trainers should always strive to make the training fun. One way to accomplish this may be to train with a parent. You may be able to kill two birds with one stone this way, since not only will both of you be getting in shape, but you'll also be able to spend some quality time together. [44,45,46]

Part III - Nutrition

"For every complicated problem there is a solution that is simple, direct, understandable, and wrong."   H.L. Mencken

This is NOT a Diet book!!! I want to make sure my readers understand I'm not trying to establish some new diet to prey off the gullible. Nor am I going to give you meal plans to follow. This chapter is instead for the purpose of dispelling myths and educating the reader. You should come away feeling much more comfortable with your knowledge of the foods you put in your mouth and perhaps, very uncomfortable with some of the foods you are currently putting into your mouth.

Which is a more common meal at your house? Your diet isn't just a way of losing weight, it's a way of eating for life.

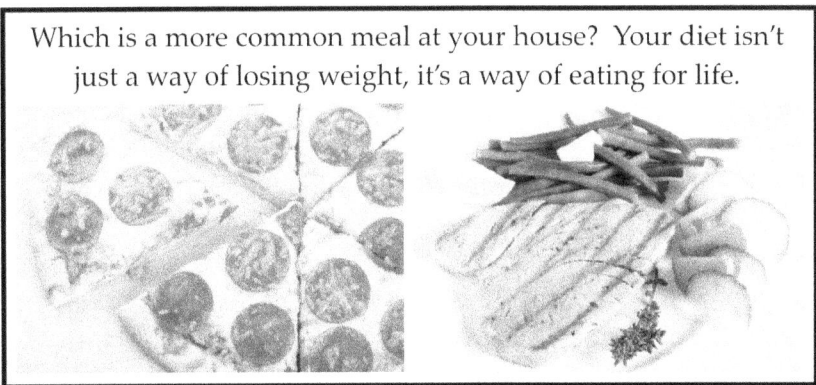

Chapter 13 – Getting Started

I've never been a fan of traditional diets. Yes, if you have the willpower, you can stay on then for a while and lose some weight. Then you'll go off the diet, and gain it all back. Without a question, the only people I have ever known who have kept their weight under control long term, have skipped the diet and just learned how to eat right.

This is even true of that friend of yours with the "fast metabolism." You know, the girl who seems to eat whatever she wants and never gains weight. Well, in reality, she probably just knows her own body and keeps her appetite under control, perhaps even without knowing it.

Very few people actually have "fast metabolisms." Your metabolic rate is almost entirely determined by the amount of lean body mass you have and by your activity level. There is some truth that fidgety people do burn more calories by nature of their constant fidgeting, but beyond that, you burn calories based on your muscle and activity.

Chances are, your friend may eat anything she wants when she wants to (when she's out in public around good food), but she probably goes home and doesn't eat the next day. Yes, she does this without really thinking about it. In that respect, she's a "natural".

I'm not saying this is the most healthy way of eating. Although many cultures throughout history did eat this way, only because their food supply was erratic and hence they ate everything in sight when it was available then perhaps went days with no food at all. But the point is, it works for her, and works a lot better than whatever many of you are doing that has caused you to end up overweight.)

It may take years, but you too can become what appears to be a "natural", once you learn how to eat right. Once you realize what certain foods really do to you, once you adjust your tastes to food that doesn't kill your goals, and once you stop using food for comfort and emotional support, you can stop the endless cycle of dieting.

No, you're not going to become a natural just from reading this book, but if you understand the concepts, start applying them every day, you can do something no other diet book will help you do: allow you to never have to worry about your weight again.

Many years ago, I struggled with my weight constantly. When I look back at all the mistakes I made, it's a little embarrassing. Now, I can pretty much manipulate my diet for any goal without even thinking about it. If I go on vacation, and eat a little too much for a week, it will only take a week after I get back to get back to my normal weight. If I'm doing a photo shoot and want to get from my normal 9% body fat, down to a ripped 6%, I almost instinctively know what to do and for how long. If I decide I want to put on a little muscle or get a little stronger, I know how to adjust my diet for that as well. But this only happened after many years of constantly adjusting my diet, logging my food intake and working on getting mentally past all my dietary hang-ups.

Keeping a Food Log

How can you do the same? First, you need to get smart about food. That's what this chapter is for, but it's also something you're going to have to learn for yourself. As with so much else in this book, much of this is different for each individual. You have to find what works for you. The first and most important part of this process is keeping an honest food log. If you don't put some time and effort into writing down EVERYTHING that goes in your mouth, you will never learn to become a "diet natural".

Whether you use computer software, a free web site, or just write it all down by hand, keeping track of what you eat, how many calories, and how many grams of protein, is the only way you will ever train yourself to eat right naturally (www.thinkingpersonsfitness.com for a great web site).

Logging your food intake has both short and long-term benefits. In the short term, you will stop fooling yourself. Yes, I know, you think you couldn't possibly lie to yourself, but you probably are. The number of mistakes I've seen clients making, that become so obvious once they start writing everything down, are too many to list.

Two examples that stand out in my memory are the guy who swore he was only eating 1200 calories a day, and couldn't figure out why he wasn't losing weight. When we logged everything, we found out he was drinking 1100 calories of Cola a day! It never even occurred to him that there were that many calories in what he was drinking.

The other example that stands out was the woman who was eating "a few almonds between meals". Almonds are healthy after all, aren't they? Turns out when she actually measured and recorded how many almonds she was eating, it added up to over a cup a day, or over 1000 extra calories!

You may say "I'd never do anything like that!" but I guarantee you are making mistakes you'd never notice otherwise.

Logging your food will enable you to really learn how to eat for the long haul. When you aren't logging your food, and you have a "cheat meal", you don't really see how bad it hurts you. When you have to log everything, you start to learn just how bad cheating can hurt you. You may think you really don't want to know, but when you know, you can choose.

For instance, I long ago gave up normal pasta and bread. It's not that I don't enjoy pasta, it's just that I know that the reality is that I can choose salmon and veggies THEN finish off with an ice cream sundae, all for the same calories as I would have eaten had I had the pasta dish and nothing else. For me, there are just better alternatives for cheating, because I KNOW what affect everything I eat will have on my diet. (I'm NOT saying an ice cream sundae is healthy, just that it's not much different than pasta)

So you can learn how to eat for yourself by keeping and analyzing your food log, or you can remain in ignorance, and struggle with your weight for the rest of your life. The choice is yours.

The point is, I'd rather teach you how to eat right, and then use exercise and slight caloric restriction to get you to the weight you want to be at. Then you can continue to eating right, but without the caloric deficit, and you will stay lean and healthy without even trying.

Diet – How we eat.

The first thing you have to understand is that "diet" is not an evil word. "Diet" simply means "way of eating". If you were trying to put on 50lbs for a belly flop competition, you'd still be on a diet, you'd just be on a weight gain diet.

The diet I recommend you follow is what I call a modern balanced diet. This is as opposed to the traditional government recommended balanced diet, which has always been much too high in processed carbohydrates, much too low in complete protein, and terribly insufficient in good fats. In this modern diet you get about 1/3rd of your calories from complex carbohydrates, 1/3rd from quality proteins, and 1/3rd from good fats. These are just approximate figures for the average person who is maintaining their weight. If you are trying to lose weight, you'll increase the protein and decrease the carbs and fats. If you are training for a marathon, then you'll increase the carbohydrates. Everyone has different needs. Some people do very well on VERY low carb diets, while others crash so badly their workouts become lazy, and overall metabolism crashes. You have to learn what works for you.

It really isn't as complicated as it sounds. All you really have to do is have a protein source and some vegetables or fruit with each meal. As you go, you will learn to adjust to what suits you best.

Chapter 14 - Macronutrients

First, we need to have a discussion of the three "macronutrients." A macronutrient as the word applies to nutrition is just a general division of the major sources of calories into three categories: Protein, Fat, and Carbohydrate. Both Proteins and Carbohydrates have 4 calories per gram. Fats have 9 calories per gram. Alcohol is distinctly different from the three basic macronutrients, and although also a source of, is not included with the other three. Alcohol has 7 calories per gram.

Protein

To say that protein is the building block of life isn't far from the truth. Protein is made up of amino acids. There are 22 amino acids that are generally considered when talking about human nutrition. Eight of them are essential. That doesn't mean that your body doesn't need the other 14, just that for the most part, your body can create the 14 non-essential amino acids by breaking down other amino acids and creating them. The eight essential amino acids (Isoleucine, Leucine, Lysine, Methionine, Phenylalanine, Threonine, Tryptophan, and Valine), must be supplied by the food we eat.

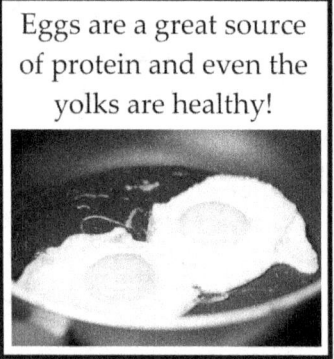

Eggs are a great source of protein and even the yolks are healthy!

To confuse the situation even further, health and fitness articles also often refer to Branched Chain Amino Acids (BCAA's), as being very important. These three amino acids are leucine, isoleucine and valine. They makeup over a 1/3 of all muscle tissue, and many studies show that supplementing with additional BCAA's will help with many different physique goals. Although this is certainly true, I feel that for most of you, concentrating on getting quality protein in adequate amounts will get you most of the way there. Worrying about things like BCAA's are for those of us with a little more time on our hands to devote to the details.

One thing you do need to worry about is the quality of the protein you are eating. I could spend a chapter just on Biological Value (BV), and Protein Efficiency Ratio (PER), but for most of you that discussion would be boring and of little value. To simplify things, let's just say that if you are consuming a variety of animal-based protein sources, the quality of protein you are getting is almost certainly sufficient, as long as you are getting adequate quantity as well.

Despite what the "experts" tell you, the most unhealthy part of this steak dinner is the potato.

On the other hand, if you are a vegetarian, or particularly a Vegan, you will have to pay much greater attention to the quality of protein you are eating, as well as the quantity. Most non-animal based protein is incomplete, meaning it doesn't contain all the necessary proteins. In this case it becomes essential that you make sure you are combining proteins that are "complimentarily incomplete". Beans and rice are an excellent example. If you only ate one of the two, you would never get the proper amino acids. However, if you eat them both, the inadequacies cancel out and you get a complete protein from the combined meal.

I won't spend too much time with the specifics required for a vegetarian diet. Suffice it to say there are better sources for this information than this book.

Protein is a controversial topic now days. There are a lot of myths flying around, and a lot of people misinterpreting it all. No, protein will not get you fit and trim on its own. No, you will not put on lean muscle just because you eat more protein. However, there are many positive aspects of this macronutrient that put it first on my list to discuss, as well as first on my list to track as well.

There's not a healthier source of protein than salmon. The most unhealthy part of this sushi is the rice!

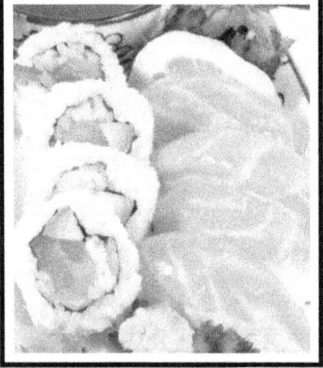

Many nutrition experts seem to base protein recommendations based on "need". As in "how much protein do you need to not get sick or not waste away. In that respect, they are correct, we don't "need" all that much. But we're not talking about what we need, we're talking about optimization. We're not just trying to keep you alive and disease free, we're also trying to optimize your health and fitness.

Besides, if we were to eliminate any of the macronutrients our body doesn't "need" we'd eliminate carbohydrates altogether, as they are the only one of the three (Protein, carbohydrates and fats) that our body does not need, either to survive or to stay healthy. I'm not talking about vitamins and minerals here, just the raw macronutrients. I'm not recommending that you give up all carbohydrates, just that they are not essential.

So, it's not that you just want to feed your body what it needs, you want to find a nutrition plan that helps you achieve and maintain the body you desire, in the fastest time possible, and maintain it with the minimum effort.

There are really two issues within the protein debate. The first is whether additional protein will help our body composition goals, and the second is whether additional protein is possibly damaging.

How Much Protein do we Need?

First, why would we ever want to consume more than the USRDA recommendation for protein? It's not as if I'm just recommending a little more protein. For most individuals I'm recommending 3 to 4 times the recommended daily allowances. Why?

The answer depends on your goals. The majority of you would like to reduce your body fat level. Notice that I say "reduce body fat", not "lose weight". It's unfortunate that all most people ever monitor is the scale. The scale only tells you how much weight you lost or gained, which can be very deceiving. Weight loss can be body fat, water, or muscle.

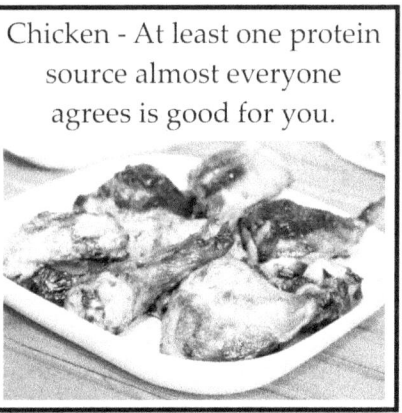

Chicken - At least one protein source almost everyone agrees is good for you.

Water weight can be a factor for two reasons. The first reason is just the daily variance in how much water you're retaining, and can be due to diet and other factors. If all you're monitoring is the scale, your body weight can go up and down several pounds from week to week. This can be discouraging, as it may seem like you're gaining weight during times when you're eating the best and working out the hardest.

Secondly, water is also a big factor in low carb diets. I'll talk about this later, but usually, the first five or so pounds of a low carb diet are really water weight, NOT body fat.

Muscle is also part of the weight loss you can see on the scale. Most conventional weight loss plans result in between 30% and 50% muscle loss. Since muscle actually burns calories 24 hours a day, and since it's the muscle that keeps things from jiggling and bouncing, the last thing ANYONE wants to do is lose muscle! And I do mean ANYONE!!

This includes the dozens of female clients I've had over the years that swear the reason they're so "thick" in the thighs is because their legs bulk up easily. It only takes a quick body fat measurement to show that this "thickness" is NOT from muscle! Remember, muscle is much denser than fat. You can take off 1 pound of fat, and add a pound of muscle, and you'll be thinner even though the scale reads the same number.

If you are one of those who still weigh the same as you did 20 years ago but you don't "look" the same, then you are a living example of the difference between fat loss and muscle loss. You've probably managed to keep your weight in check by a combination of cardio and diet. Over the years your body has gotten rid of any muscle it doesn't need (you're not using it, why would your body waste energy hauling it around), and you've ended up the same weight but flabby, and "cursed" with cellulite that you have been told is just a part of getting old.

Resistance training will minimize the amount of muscle you lose, but a big part of preventing the muscle loss while dieting is to increase your protein intake. Unfortunately, there are no real definitive studies on just how much protein is required to prevent or minimize muscle loss, but several studies have been done on very low calorie diets where nitrogen balance (a measure of muscle loss) was measured during the study. Out of the half dozen studies I've read, it can be inferred that approximately 150 grams of protein per day is necessary to minimize muscle loss.[47,48,49]

Since this would certainly be relative to the size of the person, this is where I arrive at my recommendation of 1 gram of protein per pound of ideal body weight. So, a woman, trying to get down to 130lbs should try to consume around 130 grams per day, and your average man trying to get to 180lbs should consume at least 180 grams of protein per day to try to minimize muscle loss and maximize fat loss.

Do you want more reasons why protein is beneficial while dieting? Consider the satiating effect of protein. A meal that includes protein will make you feel fuller, and remain satisfied for longer than a meal that doesn't include protein.

Or we can get even more complicated and look at the thermic effect of food. You've all heard the saying "a calorie, is a calorie, is a calorie". While this is certainly true in the laboratory, in the human body it takes an extra 10% more energy to process and utilize protein for fuel than it takes with carbs or fat. This means that you can eat 10% more calories from protein than you can from carbs or fat. That may not seem like a lot, but if the average adult reduced their calorie levels by 10%, they'd lose 22 pounds over the course of a year!

What if you're trying to put on muscle, not lose fat? Although the scientific evidence is mixed on this issue, most studies on hard training athletes show that they require at least .8 grams per pound of body weight to avoid muscle loss, and this isn't even considering those trying to build more muscle![50]

Although I'm not normally one to rely on personal observations, in light of the lack of real studies, I've never seen anyone put on a significant amount of muscle without consuming AT LEAST 1 gram per pound of body weight. Most bodybuilders or strength athletes consume even more.

Some nutritionists will tell you extra protein is not required to build muscle. Their logic is that since a pound of muscle contains only 454 grams of protein, even a very small increase in protein over the minimum requirement should allow a slow but steady gain of muscle tissue. Unfortunately, this is a case of a little knowledge being dangerous. Muscle development is a very inefficient process, with large amounts of protein turnover and nitrogen excretion necessary for the body to actually build muscle. The end-result being that much more than a pound of protein is needed to build a pound of muscle.

One note about protein consumption regardless of your goals: Your body only stores a very small amount of protein outside of muscle tissue, so anytime you go for very long without protein, your body will start to eat into the protein in your muscles, or will stop rebuilding the muscles that you worked out so hard in your last workout. So get some protein in every meal, or your body's ability to build muscle and the calorie burning effect of recovering from your workouts will both come to a halt.

How Much Protein is Safe?

What about the dangers of high protein intake? Won't your kidneys explode if you consume more than the RDA? I've even had actual MD's tell me that high protein intake can cause kidney failure.

The myth that excess protein is bad for your kidneys comes from three theories. First, weightlifters often have elevated creatinine and BUN levels, which are markers of kidney damage. Second, protein is known to be damaging to individuals with bad kidneys. Third, some have postulated that excessive protein intake causes calcium "leaching" from bones, which could lead to problems with osteoporosis. I could write pages on each of these, but to keep you from falling asleep, I'll keep it as brief as possible, as I have no intention of turning this into a text book.

Elevated creatinine and BUN levels CAN be an indicator of kidney damage, and since weightlifters will always have increased levels due to muscle microtrauma repair, and the resulting protein turnover, some doctors mistakenly assume that the high protein levels in these individual's diets are damaging their kidneys. Informed doctors will run more sophisticated tests, and these tests will almost always verify that there is no kidney damage, and that the increased Creatinine and BUN levels are simply a result of the continual muscle rebuilding.

As far as the second theory, many people also mistakenly assume that since protein is bad for people with kidney dysfunction, it must also be bad for healthy kidneys. This is really crazy, and is analogous to telling a person that since you shouldn't try to walk when your leg is broken, you should spend your life in a wheel chair even if your legs are healthy, since obviously walking is bad for your legs. An activity that is bad for a dysfunctional body part is not necessarily damaging to one that is healthy. The simple truth is that high protein diets of up to 400 grams of protein a day were used safely for the treatment of Epilepsy from the early 1900's up until the introduction of drugs to control epilepsy in the 40's and 50's, and recent studies have shown conclusively that high protein diets will not damage healthy kidneys.[51,52]

The third issue, calcium leaching, has never been proven. In fact, attempts to show that it happens have come up empty. The theory stems from the fact that excess protein intake will cause excess calcium excretion in the Urine. However, studies actually show that subjects with higher protein intakes have INCREASED bone density. Yes, this is probably from many other factors, however the fact remains, when combined with proper exercise, excess protein helps bone density.

So there you have it. Add some healthy protein to each and every meal, and you'll feel fuller, lose more fat, and maintain or increase that metabolically active and firm muscle.

Protein Shakes

You don't get enough protein to optimize your progress toward reaching your goals. Yes, I can make this statement without knowing anything about your diet or your goals. I've almost never seen someone who didn't benefit from more protein in their diet. The reasons are listed earlier.

However, it's hard to get more protein and many of my clients struggle to get even close to my recommendations (mainly due to bad dietary habits they have yet to shake). Protein powder mixed into a simple drink or smoothie is an easy, low cal and inexpensive way to do it. Many people say they think protein powder is too expensive, but on a $ per gram of protein basis, protein powder is about as economical as it comes.

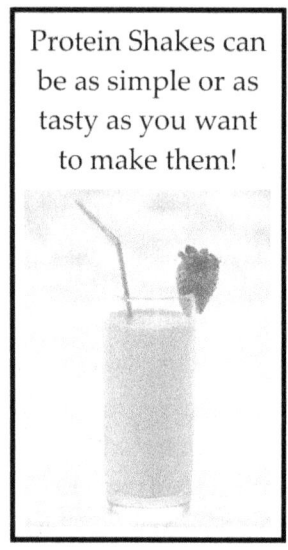

Protein Shakes can be as simple or as tasty as you want to make them!

You do not need to get complicated with this. Even the simplest products work just fine. Many companies will try to make a big deal about the type of protein. I do recommend whey protein (a milk based protein) most of the time as it is the cheapest, easiest to mix quality protein available. But for the most part, the type of protein is really irrelevant. The manufacturers will point to the rates of digestion of each type (hydrolysate for quicker absorption after working out or casein before bed for slower digestion) but the truth is the rate of digestion is irrelevant once other ingredients are added. For instance, in the evening, adding a little flax oil (Omega3's) to your protein shake will slow digestion far more than using casein. Some prefer Soy protein for some supposed magical hormonal benefits that never really materialize in studies, but there's really no reason to obsess over either the type or brand of protein powder you use.

The only item you really need to look for is what else is added, how does it mix, and how does it taste.

Many products add sugar or other stuff to make it a "Meal Replacement Shake." There's nothing wrong with that but just watch out that you're not getting stuff you don't need (like extra calories). As far as taste and mixability, that's a matter of personal taste. I recommend some brands I like on my web site. You may have to try a couple brands to find one you really like, although I find most people will like just about any brand once they get used to it. Don't give up just because you didn't like the first shake you made. With time, it will start to taste much better.

I try to stick with simple flavors (vanilla and chocolate), and then add ingredients to the shakes for taste or to make a full meal out of them.

A protein shake can be as simple as mixing a scoop and a half into 8 oz of water in a shaker bottle to pour over your cereal in place of milk (to avoid the extra sugar in the milk), or as complicated as a smoothie with berries, yogurt and flax oil, or a mocha drink with chocolate powder, espresso, and sugar free kahlua flavored syrup. These last two are particularly tasty. Even people who hate most healthy foods will usually like these.

Some people try to stay away from artificial sweeteners. Each brand of shake uses something different as a sweetener. Check around to find one that's right for you. Some are unsweetened, so you can put in whatever you desire. Just because you don't like the taste of one brand is no reason to give up on protein shakes altogether.

Protein Bars

Yes, we're all busy. REALLY busy! Sometimes eating right is darn near impossible. Although there's no real substitute for a good healthy meal, there's certainly something better than a candy bar out of the snack machine: Protein Bars. As with protein shakes, protein bars can be a valuable tool in your nutrition toolbox.

What makes a protein bar any better than a candy bar? Well, to be quite honest, in many cases, not much. You've probably seen a million ads for healthy snack bars: Nutri-this, Healthy-that. These really are just glorified candy bars. No, they probably don't have as

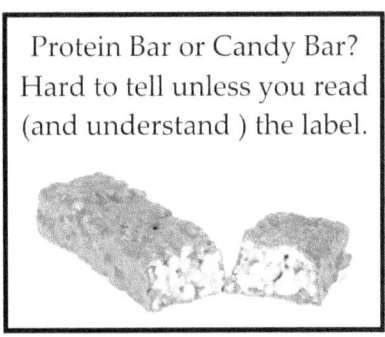

Protein Bar or Candy Bar? Hard to tell unless you read (and understand) the label.

much bad fat in them, but since they're also completely lacking any good fat or protein and are high in processed carbs, they produce a tremendous sugar rush. Eat one, and your insulin levels will skyrocket for half an hour, then plummet causing even sharper hunger pains than you had a half hour before.

Some of the so-called protein bars on the market are not much better. With only a little low quality protein, and lots of sugar, you have to be careful what you buy. That's where the label comes in right? Well, kind of. Unfortunately, many manufacturers play a funny game with the labels as well. You see, it's almost impossible to make a reasonably tasty bar with decent texture and moisture without carbs (think beef jerky).

Pretty much every protein bar uses "sugar alcohols" to help with taste, sweetness, and texture, and the use of these sugar alcohols can make the labels a little confusing (see the sugar alcohols topic under the carbohydrates section.

So, what happens when we walk into the health food store and look at the rack of Health Bars? First we find one with some protein. At least 20 grams if not 30. It should also be good quality protein. Whey, Casein, and maybe some Soy, but if it says gelatin near the top of the list, stay away. Gelatin is a filler protein. Technically it's still a protein, but it has near zero biological value.

Then we look at the fat. A little fat isn't a bad thing. It slows digestion and keeps you from getting hungry as fast. I'd stay away from any bar with much saturated fat or any trans-fats.

Now what about carbs? Most of the manufacturers of low carb bars count on the fact that you'll look at the total carb count and be happy that it says 4 grams. We know that's not true because it would chew like a piece of beef jerky. You could add up the grams of carbs and protein and multiply that number by 4. Then you could multiply the grams of fat by 9 and add that to the other number. Subtract the number of calories on the label by this number, then you have the number of calories of "hidden carbs".

Since this is a little complicated to do with every bar you look at, I recommend you just find the highest protein content with the lowest total calories and give it a try for taste and digestion. Unless of course you are trying to add weight, in which case you might be looking for higher calories.

The healthiest bars are not necessarily the lowest calories. There are some very tasty bars out there that are low in sugar alcohols, but have added sugar and fat for taste. They are certainly better than candy bars, and if weight gain isn't a problem for you, these are a great alternative.

I am still looking for a great pre/post-workout bar. I'd like it to have plenty of fast digesting sugars, along with plenty of protein, with no sugar alcohols or fat. Sometimes taking an after workout shake with you is just not convenient. A bar like this would be great. I haven't found one yet. Send me an email or post to my forum if you know of a good one.

What bar do I recommend? I've given up on this question. Everyone seems to like a different bar. The bars I love, you might hate. Besides, it depends on what you're looking for: Energy with some protein, super low carbs with less taste, or a balance. You can go to my web site (www.thinkingpersonsfitness.com) and you'll find a of couple different bars. They all have quality protein, and I think they all taste decent.

Just be careful! These are not zero calories! You can't just eat them all the time and think you're still controlling your diet. If it's a 200 calorie bar, you need to subtract 200 calories of food from your diet for that day. I recommend that most people plan their diets with one "planned snack". This can be eaten at any time when you just can't make it to the next planned meal. That's a great use for a protein bar.

Carbohydrates

Very simply put, carbohydrates are cheap fuel. A food high in carbohydrates may contain other nutrients as well, but whether a carbohydrate contains primarily starches, or sugars, the end result is the same, the only use your body has for them is in supplying energy or being converted to fat for later use as energy.

Carbohydrates are the only macronutrient that is NOT essential. This means you do not need them to survive, unlike fats and proteins.

What's the difference between white bread, rice, pasta and table sugar? From your body's point of view, not much!!

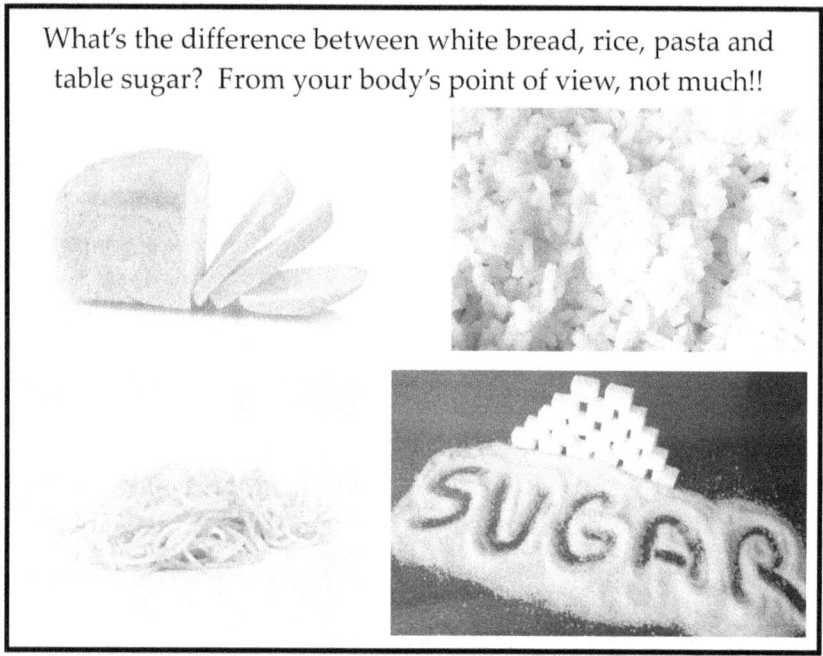

Americans eat too many carbohydrates for their lifestyles! This is a simple truth that it is hard to get around regardless of your personal nutritional opinions. Our dietary habits have changed for the worse over the last 30 years in many ways, but the large amounts of carbohydrates in almost every meal we eat is excessive given our sedentary lifestyles. Much of our eating habits are a carryover from many generations ago when a much larger amount of cheap energy was needed to fuel our daily activities.

Also, since the advent of federally subsidizing corn, high fructose corn syrup (sugar) has become so cheap that it's in just about everything. If you are interested in the story behind the poisoning of the American people by their own government, as well as a lot of other interesting information, I highly recommend the book Fat Land.[53]   There is a review on my web site as well as a link.

Food Production and Civilization

A little history lesson: One of the defining characteristics of an advanced civilization is that a few people can supply food for many. Thousands of years ago, our ancestors were just like any other animal on the planet: each individual had to supply its own food. No one had time for other pursuits, as food was the constant primary concern.   As our society moved to an agricultural society, one person was able to supply food for several people.   Once the ratio of food consumers to food suppliers grew to about 10 to 1 modern society was able to start developing, as the majority of individuals were able to concentrate on tasks other than supplying food. Currently in the US, an average farmer produces enough food for over 130 people. This allows us A LOT of time for activities other than producing food.

The problem is, a long time ago farmers learned that the best way to grow enough food (calories) for a lot of people was to grow very simple crops: crops that contain calories and not much more than calories.   Examples would be simple carbohydrates, like grain, corn, potatoes, rice, etc. As an added benefit, since these crops had very little in the way of color or nutrients, they could be grown on a smaller amount of land where the nutrient density of the soil was not a big factor.

A hundred years ago, this wasn't such a bad thing since we didn't have many of today's horrible dietary habits, and we spent all day doing manual labor (therefore requiring more calories for energy). Today, however, the extra energy we get from the simple carbohydrates that are still so plentiful in our diets, just get stored as body fat.

The Solution

The simple fact of modern life is that if you want to greatly simplify the task of maintaining your weight, you MUST minimize your intake of bread, pasta, rice, potato and of course, all sugary drinks. We are no longer an agrarian society participating in manual labor. Most of us are completely sedentary throughout the day and therefore do not need high levels of carbohydrates to sustain our energy. Additionally, carbohydrates are addictive. The more candy you eat, the more you want.

The bulk of your carbohydrates should come from vegetables and fruit. Moreover, those with high water content, such as cucumbers, grapefruit, tomatoes, cantaloupe, strawberries, watermelon and even vegetable soups, will fill you up nicely. By the way, numerous studies have conclusively proven that the quarter of the population eating the most vegetables gets half the cancer of the quarter eating the least!

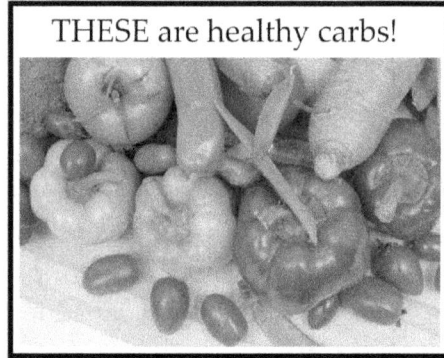

THESE are healthy carbs!

As an additional benefit, vegetables are high in fiber. Fiber is best known for keeping us "regular", but it has also been shown to cause weight loss all on its own. That's right, when you increase your fiber consumption (through eating more vegetables), you will probably lose a couple pounds without doing anything else.

Perhaps one of the biggest mistakes I see in even a "healthy" family diet, is the need to have bread and potatoes in every dinner. In fact, this is so ingrained in the American way of eating, that some people look at a dinner consisting of meat and vegetables as being a bit weird. Try to convince most Americans that the bread and potatoes in the evening, right at the time they DON'T need extra energy, is a bad thing, and they'll just look at you funny. Problem is, as much as you might think this type of meal is "normal," eliminating the bread and potatoes (or pasta) is probably the easiest single step you can take to maintaining your waistline.

Zero Carb or Atkins Diets

Why don't I generally recommend the zero carb diets? I think we can safely say that the low/zero carb craze is certainly one of the biggest diet fads of the last decade. Certainly one of the most controversial.

On the one, side you have Atkins and others claiming that low carb diets are healthy and will allow you to lose far more weight than any other type of diet and that you can eat all the fat you want as long as you eliminate the carbs.

On the other, side you have the "establishment" with their food pyramid saying low carb diets don't result in greater weight loss than conventional diets, and the high fat content will cause you to drop dead of a heart attack.

Who's right? Well, actually they're both right (and wrong). Low or no carb diets will not magically cause you to lose weight while you eat all the fat you can eat, but they also won't kill you.

Carbs and Your Heart

"But fat is bad for our hearts" you say. Well that's a topic for an entirely separate discussion, and to cover it adequately would take a chapter and another hundred references, but suffice it to say, the long established but never proven link between high fat diets and heart disease is now slowly being eroded.

As an example, the indigenous Eskimo population of Alaska eats a diet which is almost 75% saturated fats for much of the year yet has a very low instance of heart disease. Take these same Eskimos and feed them a typical "healthy" American diet high in carbs and low in saturated fats, and they start dropping of heart disease just like the rest of us. Despite the fact that Americans are eating less fat, and significantly less saturated fat than ever before, our death rate due to heart disease is RISING.

I clearly remember an incident from a few years ago that really puzzled me. The news was on the TV in the studio and out of the corner of my mind I heard the reporter talking about a study done on low carb diets. I don't remember the particular details of the study, but what I will never forget was the researcher (who obviously started out to prove that low carb diets didn't work), reported that study participants actually LOWERED traditional indicators of potential heart disease (bad cholesterol, triglycerides, blood pressure, etc). He then stated something to the effect of "But we must have made an error somewhere, as everyone KNOWS that high fat diets are bad for the heart". This very prejudiced researcher couldn't even objectively view his own data, such was the strength of his previously held (and erroneous) beliefs.

Zero Carbs and Miracle Weight Loss

So if the above is correct, and Adkins was right about a low carb, high fat diet being healthy, what was he wrong about? We know all about the miraculous weight loss that proponents of low carb diets claim. Right? Wrong! In reality they don't exist. Nothing, I repeat NOTHING violates the first law of thermodynamics: In any closed system, the energy in must equal the energy out plus the energy accumulated within the system. In other words, regardless of what ANY "expert" tells you, the only conceivable method of weight loss is to expend more energy than you consume. Atkins, and the zero carb proponents cannot offer any explanation as to how their methods break this LAW of thermodynamics. They will cite the fact that when you're on a zero carb diet your body might excrete energy as ketones in your urine. However, it has been scientifically proven that this loss is insignificant in the scheme of things.[54]

"So what about the studies" you say. Yes, Atkins does have a few studies showing extra weight loss at the start of a low carb diet. However, these studies all suffer the same flaw: they ignore water loss. You see, when you deplete the body of glycogen (carbs), you also lose water. Glycogen is stored in the body attached to water in a 1 to 4 ratio. What that means is that for every gram of carbohydrate you lose, you also lose 4 grams of water. It is well known that at the start of a carb depletion diet, the average person will lose 4 to 15 lbs of water.[55,56,57] Water that you will eventually gain back, and that does not contribute to fat loss (the real weight loss target).

What about all the real world evidence? All those testimonials? Well, zero carb diets used to have one thing going for them. It used to be very hard to find food with no carbs. How much bacon or beef jerky can you eat before you just can't eat any more bacon and beef jerky? There used to be absolutely nothing in the snack machine at work that didn't have carbs. People

> The reason zero carb diets can work is the same reason the grapefruit diet can work - Just how much grapefruit (or bacon) can you eat before you just don't want to eat another piece?

lost weight because they were lowering their calorie intake without knowing it. I say "used to" because now with the advent of low carb and no carb food in every grocery store and snack machine, it has become easy to overeat even on a no carb diet. People who used to find low carb diets useful, are now finding they don't lose weight like they used to.

If you think about it, the fact that people are using these diets off and on for years should tell you all you need to know: A diet isn't effective if you just gain the weight back again. Since all these diets are temporary solutions, and not permanent healthy changes, they will always fail in the long run.

This is NOT to say a low fat, high carb diet is the way to go. The previous discussion was only in reference to ZERO carb diets. As discussed, Americans do eat way too many processed carbs for our lifestyle. These carbs (bread, pasta, sugars, potatoes, rice, etc.) have next to zero nutritional value, provide too much energy for our sedentary lifestyles, and spike our insulin levels causing us to be hungry sooner after a meal. This insulin spike may actually be responsible for our rise in heart disease as it is theorized to result in hardening of the arteries. This blood sugar spike doesn't occur when fat is eaten along with the carbs, which would be a possible explanation for American rise in heart disease: we've increased our carb consumption at the same time we've tried to eliminate fats from our diets. Yes, all those fat-free foods you've been eating may very well be killing you!

While we're talking about carbohydrates, I'm going to venture off on a small but related tangent. You've heard me use the terms, sugars, processed carbohydrates, and even "White carbohydrates" as terms for the types of carbs you should be avoiding. There are two properties that a "bad" carb has that a good carb doesn't: first is the lack of nutrients in bad carbs. It's no coincidence that most bad carbs lack any sort of color (hence "white carbs"). White bread, rice, potatoes, they're all pretty much sugar in a different package, just calories and nothing more.

The other quality bad carbohydrates have to a greater or lesser extent is how fast they are turned into sugar once in your body, and hence how fast your blood sugar spikes.

Glycemic Index

There's a term for that and it's called Glycemic Index. It's one term I never thought I'd see become popular in the media and weight loss world. Unlike many other junk terms thrown around on commercials, Glycemic Index really can be useful. However, it's also misused and overused.

Glycemic Index (GI) is defined as the increase in blood sugar levels that occur in the body after a certain carbohydrate-rich food is eaten. As a standard, white bread is defined as a GI of 100, and is considered High GI. The lower the GI, the less that particular food spikes your blood sugar.

Why is blood sugar so important? Because spiking your blood sugar causes your body to release insulin in order to process (and store) the sugar. These repeated, rapid insulin releases are the primary causes of Type II diabetes or general insulin resistance, and therefore is a major factor in obesity. Blood sugar is also, contrary to popular opinion, one of the primary factors in heart disease. Yes, perhaps a much greater factor than dietary fat intake![58,59,60,61,62]

So how can we use Glycemic Index, and how is it being misused? In a very broad sense, if we restrict our carbohydrate intake to low GI foods, we are less likely to experience any form of insulin resistance, and therefore reduce the risk of weight gain. High GI foods will also cause us to be hungry again very soon after eating, since they are absorbed so fast, and low GI carbs will a help keep us from eating again as soon since your blood sugar will stay regulated longer.

The problem with the way the diet industry is currently using the Gylcemic Index is that they are defining "Healthy Carbs" by the Glycemic Index. If you go back to our initial definition of what makes a carb "bad", you'll notice blood sugar response is only half of it. Just because an over processed, nutrient depleted food has a low GI, doesn't make it healthy. Also, what is "Low GI", and whose

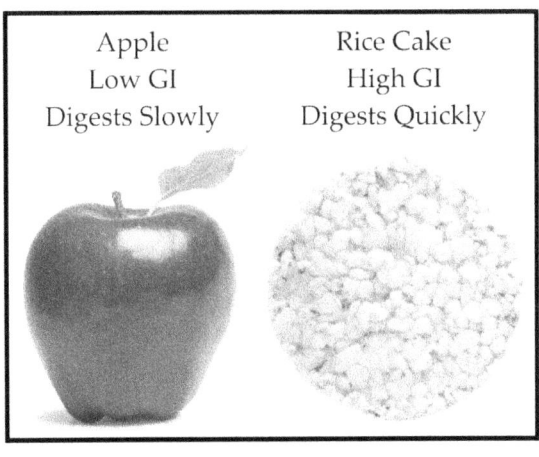

Apple	Rice Cake
Low GI	High GI
Digests Slowly	Digests Quickly

definition of low are we using? I've looked at some of these Low GI meals and wonder exactly how the manufacturers are coming up with their definition.

Another misuse of Glycemic Index is that it's really not the GI of the individual food that counts: it's the GI of the entire meal that matters. If all you're worried about is the blood sugar spike, dipping a piece of white bread in a vat of lard will reduce the GI to a very low level. But is it really healthy? The white bread still contains nothing of nutritional value. It's still just empty calories, and lots of them.

Where GI becomes useful is when comparing individual foods for their ability to fill you up and not spike your blood sugar. In other words, an Apple (GI of 38) is a better snack than a banana (GI of 56) or rice cakes (GI of 88). Lima beans (32) are better than mashed potatoes (70). You could check this by using a blood sugar meter like a diabetic uses. You'd take readings every 15 minutes after eating the food, but I don't recommend doing this at home (yes, I've done it). The difference becomes pretty obvious if you've ever noticed how an apple will keep the hunger away for quite a while, and after a banana you'll be hungry again in half an hour.

However, GI is not really that useful on a day to day basis. Understanding the theory is what will help us to avoid sugary foods, white bread, white rice, or white potatoes. However, we could have also found the same information by looking at the fiber content of each food. In most cases it's the fiber that makes a carbohydrate low GI, and fiber is also one of the factors I would use to classify a food as "healthy".

Take bread for example: you can pretty much tell whether a bread is healthy by its fiber content. Although someone could certainly put fiber back into plain white bread, no one does. In fact, the opposite is true. Most "wheat bread" is simply dyed white bread, and is no healthier than plain white bread. It may be fortified, but really does not contain any of the natural fibers or nutrients that were in the grain before it was processed. If you are looking for a "healthy" bread, you are much better off looking for a "whole grain" bread, and then checking the fiber content. I look for at least 3-4 grams of fiber per slice.

So, yes, GI is a useful concept, but only if you are talking about individual foods in their natural form. Old fashioned oatmeal may have a GI of 48, but Cheerios (despite the manufacturer's health claims) has a GI of 78 (processed in your body almost like sugar). Pizza Hut Supreme Pizza has a GI of 33 (because of all the fat that slows digestion), but that doesn't mean it's good for your weight loss plan!

A Simpler Way

Don't let the last topic confuse you or scare you away. You really can keep it pretty simple. Just confine your carbs almost entirely to fruits and vegetables. Many people will try to complicate things by telling you certain fruits are too high in sugar, and although this may be true to some extent, the fact remains, I've NEVER seen anyone get fat on fruits and vegetables!

In fact, several studies have shown that eating an apple before a meal will actually result in fewer total calories being consumed (including the apple) than if the apple wasn't eaten. Yes, even though apples have a lot of sugar in them, the high fiber content satiates enough to make a big difference. Yes, broccoli before a meal would probably work even better, but who's going to carry around broccoli?

Sugar Alcohols

You will find sugar alcohols in just about every "health food" on the market today. It's not really a true sugar, but it tastes like one to some extent. What's interesting about them from a food producer's point of view is that sometimes the manufacturers don't have to count it as a carb. This is derived from the fact that it won't affect blood sugar levels to any significant extent in a diabetic.

The low carb food manufacturers use this as an excuse not to list them. They say that if it won't affect ketosis (arguable since the liver still converts sugar alcohols to glucose in limited amounts), it won't affect a low-carber's diet. This depends on the type of sugar alcohol. You still need to look at the total calories.

Another problem with sugar alcohols is that for many people they really mess up their digestive process if consumed too often. I won't go into the nasty details, but if you buy some protein bars and the next day have issues, you know the culprit. This is one of the reasons I recommend limiting yourself to one protein bar per day. Some people have no issues at all, and some will smell up a room 15 minutes after eating any at all.

The following chart shows some of the common sugar alcohols along with their relative sweetness, and number of calories actually absorbed. As a rule of thumb, the less calories absorbed, the worse the digestive issues. I have read that erythritol does not have any digestive side effects, and I have used it as a sugar substitute with some success, but I am not sure everyone will find it as side effect free as some do.[63]

Name	Sweetness	Calories (kcal/g)
Sucrose (sugar)	1.0	4.0
Arabitol	0.7	0.2
Erythritol	0.8	0.2
Glycerol	0.6	4.3
Isomalt	0.5	2.0
Lactitol	0.4	2.0
Maltitol	0.9	2.1
Mannitol	0.5	1.6
Sorbitol	0.6	2.6
Xylitol	1.0	2.4

This chart is probably more complicated than most of you want to get, but I included it so you'd be more aware of what the ingredients are in the foods you are eating.

I am not going to discuss other sugar substitutes, either natural (Stevia) or manmade (Saccharin, Aspartame, Sucralose), as all they do is add sweetness without calories. I'll leave the conspiracy theories on whether they are bad for you to others.

Fat

Fat is a term used for a broad range of compounds also often referred to as Fatty Acids, or Lipids. Like Proteins, these compounds are essential for life. While most types of fat can be manufactured inside our bodies from proteins and carbohydrates, some fats are considered "essential fatty acids". These fats can't be made by our bodies, and must be present in our diets. These are the Omega-3 and Omega-6 fatty acids. Our diets generally contain all of the Omega-6 fatty acids we need, but our modern diets have pretty much processed out any Omega-3's. The studies you see touting the amazing health benefits of Omega-3's are a statement of how important these fatty acids are and how horribly deficient our diets are in Omega-3's.

Eat fat to lose fat!

This is a statement that some people find outrageous, but to some degree, it's true. Fat has gotten a bad reputation for two reasons. First, it's fat! It's the same thing we're trying to get OUT of our bodies. Why wouldn't we want to drop it from our diets? Secondly and a little more scientifically, fat contains over twice the calories of protein or carbohydrates. Eat a pound of fat and you will be eating almost 4100 calories. If you eat a pound of white bread you'll only be consuming a little over 1800 calories. How could fats NOT be bad?

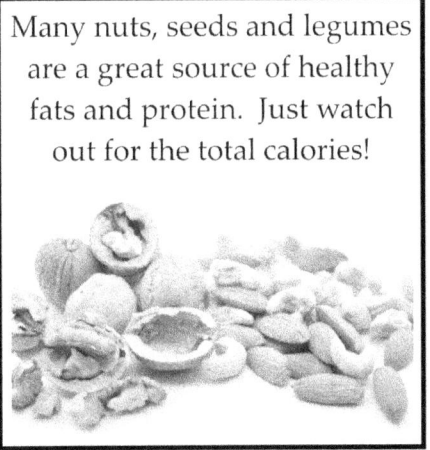

Many nuts, seeds and legumes are a great source of healthy fats and protein. Just watch out for the total calories!

To some extent, this is true. It is very easy to eat a lot of calories from fat, and as with sugar, it's easy to hide a lot of calories of fat in various foods. The calorie content of a fast food hamburger is much higher than a sandwich from a sub shop. That's the reason Jared can lose so much weight eating nothing but subs. It's not that subs are a good diet food, they aren't, but the lack of fat makes a big difference.

However, it doesn't always work that way. Many times, when all the fat is taken out of a certain food, the resulting product is so unsatiating that you're hungry again very quickly after eating it. On top of that, foods without much fat generally taste pretty bad, and many manufacturers make up for it by just adding more sugar or other refined carbs. Many of the "low fat" snack foods are this way. If you only ate one, you'd be ok, but it's next to impossible to eat only one. They are just so terribly unfilling because of all the carbs with no fat to slow down digestion.

Why Fats are Essential

However, the really bad part about trying to avoid dietary fats is the fact that many healthy fats are necessary to your body for many reasons: regulating hormonal production, improving immune function, lowering total cholesterol, lubricating joints, and providing the basics for healthy hair, nails and skin. Unlike carbohydrates, which are not necessary for staying alive, fats are very critical to not only your long term health, but also short term fitness. In fact some fats are so helpful (and so lacking in a modern American diet), that consumption of these fats will actually result in weight loss in certain individuals!

The singular distinction you must be aware of is the difference between healthy "good" fats and dangerous "bad" fats. Good fats are monounsaturated fats like olive, peanut and canola oil, avocados, all natural peanut butter and nuts; and omega-3 fats like salmon, tuna, flax seeds and mackerel. Bad fats are partially hydrogenated fats (killers!), and trans fats, as well as ALL fried foods. Almost anything you buy in a box or bag has bad fats and no good fats.

Saturated Fats – Not all bad

Many people would put all saturated fats in the bad category as well, however any studies showing a link between saturated fat and heart disease have failed to remove many other factors that we now know will greatly affect heart health.[64] Many new studies are showing a lot of difference between types of saturated fats. [65]

There is still a lot of conflicting studies on this, but I will go out on a limb and state that 20 years from now, it will be common knowledge that, for the most part, if it's fat that comes directly from nature (yes, even animal fats), it's ok. If it's processed in any way, you should probably stay away from it.

The REAL Bad Fats

Probably the best example of this is deep frying. There is probably no worse process you can do to fat than heat it to a high temperature. Every fat has a specific temperature at which it starts to break down into some very nasty stuff, but regardless of the type of oil used, once you've heated it to deep frying temperature, bad stuff happens. Certain fast food restaurants would like you to believe their fried foods are healthier because they are fried in vegetable oil instead of lard. The problem is, once ANY oil is heated to over 350 degrees for more than 10 minutes, it then has the nutritional value of used motor oil!!

> If it comes in a bag or a box, it probably has plenty of "bad" fats.

Deep-fried food is probably the only food I can say beyond doubt should be eliminated from your diet! Almost every food, whether it's steak, chocolate or red wine, has some nutrients to contribute. But one thing is absolute: fried foods are bad for you. Potato chips, French fries, onion rings, breaded chicken strips and all the rest of the deep-fried junk are pregnant with the worst kinds of fats and calories. If you're trying to lose weight and/or reduce fat, simply eliminate fried foods completely from your diet.

I know, easier said than done. I'll be the first to admit, it was MUCH easier to eliminate processed carbs from my diet than it was to eliminate fried foods. To be honest, I haven't totally succeeded. There are times when I just CRAVE some french fries or chicken strips.

There is some debate that fried food may even be cancerous. Frying carbohydrates produces a known carcinogen, and some also theorize that the changes in the fat molecule may be cancerous as well.

The bottom line is that your body needs good fats (especially omega-3's which our diets are deficient in) and will revolt if you attempt to abstain from them – and absolutely does not need bad fats. If that weren't enough, adding a little good fat to a meal will satiate you for longer since it will take your body longer to process the meal. This means it will be longer until you're hungry again.

Omega 3 Fatty Acids – Fish Oil

On the topic of good fats, fish oil or Omega 3 fatty acids are the kings. You absolutely MUST supplement with Fish Oil!! If you are not, you are missing out on the single biggest and easiest thing you can do for your health!! I'm not joking!

It seems everywhere I look lately, someone has got something to say about Omega 3's. Maybe that doesn't ring a bell, but maybe you've seen something on TV about Fish Oils (same thing), or Bad Fats/Good Fats (Omega 3's would be the good fats).

Some of the facts behind Omega 3's and the benefits of supplementing them:

- The modern American diet contains only a fraction of the Omega 3's that our ancestor's diets had.

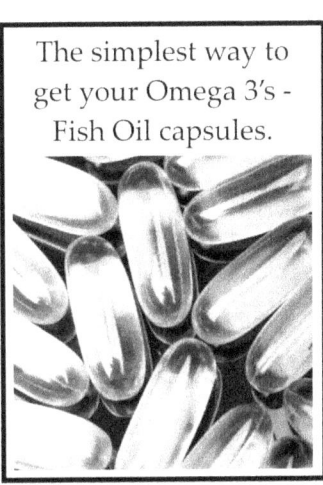

The simplest way to get your Omega 3's - Fish Oil capsules.

- Omega 3's aren't a magic supplement. They're a fat. Just like saturated fat, polyunsaturated fats, etc.
- When our livestock was free range (wandered the fields eating grass), it had an almost ideal amount of Omega 3's. Now that our livestock is grain fed, our beef, chicken, eggs, etc. contain almost no Omega 3's
- You can get Omega 3's from Flax Oil, Fish oil from capsules or bottled Cod Liver oil (yes, your Grandma was right about the Cod Liver Oil!!), salmon, and from livestock raised on small free-range farms. Fish Oil is by far the best source. Flax Oil and seeds do not contain the specific type of Omega 3 that your body really needs.
- Most people eat more than 100grams of fat a day, hence taking 1gram of omega 3's does next to nothing. Most studies done on Omega 3's use dosages between 5 and 20 grams a day (1 gram = 1000mg = One fish oil capsule). Most supplement companies recommend one or two grams a day on their product labels. This is a legal and marketing issue, and has nothing to do with the actual amount we need to take.

Some well Proven Benefits of Increasing Omega 3's
- Heart Health - 50% less chance of a primary cardiac arrest than people whose daily menu does not contain these fatty acids.
- Weight loss – Individuals fed supplemental Omega 3's lose a small amount of weight without changing anything else about their diets or exercise routine.

- Rheumatoid Arthritis – patients suffering from this disease showed decreased symptoms and a reduced need for medication
- Hair and Skin health – Omega 3's have been shown to reduce the effects of aging on skin. Hair of people who supplement with Omega 3's is healthier and fuller.
- May help prevent depression.
- Decreased menstrual symptoms among women.
- Prevention and treatment of kidney diseases.
- Improved ratio of "good/bad" cholesterol.
- Increased Testosterone production – Important for men trying to gain muscle and women trying to lose stubborn lower body fat (also increases libido in both sexes)
- Increased Insulin sensitivity – helps prevent Type II diabetes (or reduce its effects)
- Decrease inflammatory effects of training or injury.

Remember, this is just FOOD. It's not some magical drug. All of these benefits are subtle and long term. You may not really notice a big difference right away, but the facts behind the benefits of these fats are still there. I don't care how much fish you eat. Most of it is corn fed, and doesn't have the omega 3 content it should. You still need to supplement.

The newer fish oil capsules are reasonably priced, very concentrated, have no aftertaste, and have been tested for heavy metal content (Mercury, etc.).

Make sure you stick with concentrated Omega 3 or fish oil supplements. Many companies are trying to market Omega3-6-9 supplements, however, most of us already get enough Omega6-9 fats in our diets. Supplementing further with these will, at best be a waste of money, and at worst, may have pro-inflammatory effects that counteracts the effects of the Omega 3's.

If you do nothing else after reading this book, go to my web site and order yourself some fish oil capsules!!

Chapter 15 - Nutrient Timing:

Whether or not you want to worry about nutrient timing, or when to eat which foods is up to you. It's one of those topics that many people just don't want to be bothered with, and that is understandable, however even if you are one of those people, having a basic awareness of how what you eat when can affect your health and fitness goals, may help you make small but important decisions.

There are many reasons to be concerned about the timing of the foods you eat. But regardless of what type of nutrient we are speaking of, the primary reason is that it always helps to give your body what it needs, when it needs it. Your body is not very efficient at storing nutrients such as proteins, and if you feed your body carbohydrates for energy when you don't need the energy, it will just be converted to fat. However, if you feed your body carbs at the right time, it can use them to fuel your activities much more efficiently or help you recover quicker from a tough workout.

Break-Fast

Let's start with breakfast. It's almost cliché at this point, but breakfast really is the most important meal of the day. If our eating habits weren't so rooted in tradition, it would be taken much more seriously than it is, and our food choices would be a lot different as well.

Breakfast doesn't have to be much different from other meals, but most of us do tend to eat different foods at this time of day. Most of us either eat a breakfast that consists almost entirely of carbohydrates, or one almost entirely made up of fats. Either one doesn't do you any favors.

Although breakfast is certainly one time of day when the body can use carbs for fuel, the massive quantity of carbs most people eat for breakfast just results in a massive sugar shock that will leave you lethargic mid way through the morning. Cereal, milk, Orange juice, toast, jam, etc. are all made almost entirely of sugar.

Cereal – High Carb Breakfasts

Common cereals are perhaps the biggest offenders. Despite the labels, your body treats them just like a bowl full of sugar. It's nice to finally see the FDA cracking down on some manufacturer's health claims, but we've got a long way to go. The cereal aisle is basically one big "morning candy" isle, and that includes most of the popular "healthy" brands.

There are a few brands that are reasonably healthy. You can recognize them by the fact that they contain some reasonable amount of fiber, as well as protein and healthy fats. These "granola like" cereals do tend to be pretty high in calories, so you need to make sure you measure out how much you are eating. Some of the "bran" type cereals are decent as well, as long as they're not covered in sugar. REAL oatmeal may also be good when combined with healthy fats and protein (not the processed kind in a package).

The next culprit is the milk we put on top our cereal. While many consider it a healthy source of protein and nutrients, modern processed milk is almost entirely sugar, with only a small amount of quality protein. Since most of us are accustomed to skim or 2%, our milk contains almost no healthy fat as well.

A bowl of most of the commonly considered "healthy" cereals along with skim milk will send your body into a state of sugar shock not much different from candy or sugar filled soda. I've tested this myself. It's pretty dramatic.

I will admit that cereal is a very practical breakfast. Most of us don't want to take the time to cook anything in the morning. My personal solution is one of the healthy cereals I mentioned above along with a densely mixed vanilla protein shake (protein powder and water). The fiber, protein, and healthy fats in this breakfast will totally blunt the blood sugar reaction and cause you to feel satiated for much longer. It may take some time to get used to the taste, but once you do, you'll never miss the milk.

Juice – Just Sugar Water

The third big culprit in American breakfasts is fruit juice, or specifically orange juice. We've been told for so long that these are healthy for us that it's hard for us to even imagine that the juice producers have been lying to us for this long. The hard facts are that turning a fruit into a juice results in most of the good stuff being removed and only the sugar remaining. Fruit juice is not fruit, it's effectively just sugar water. It's not much better than regular sugar filled sodas. If you insist on drinking OJ at breakfast, consider it a treat, but don't fool yourself into thinking it's healthy. Yes, there are a few vitamins but most of them are fortified, which means it's no different from what you'd get in a multi-vitamin, only with tons of unnecessary sugar and calories.

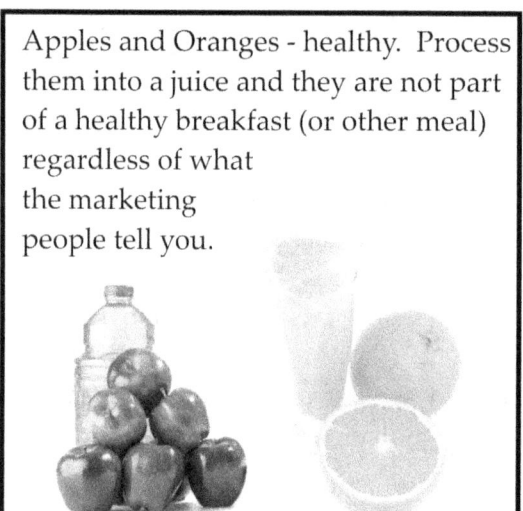

Apples and Oranges - healthy. Process them into a juice and they are not part of a healthy breakfast (or other meal) regardless of what the marketing people tell you.

A current advertisement for one very popular children's drink states that it has "one third less sugar than soda!" Which to my mind, is sort of like saying "One third less cyanide than rat poison!" STAY AWAY from sugar filled drinks of any kind!

High Fat Breakfasts

The next category of breakfast is the high fat breakfast. Eggs, bacon, sausage, etc.etc. There's nothing wrong with these foods in and of themselves if you choose the right brands, but the problem is they are so high in calories from all the fats, that it's hard to start off a day where you plan to only eat 1700 calories, if your first meal contains 1200.

Personally, I prefer to get most of my fats at night when the satiating effect will keep me full through the night. I like to get a little bit of healthy fat with my morning meal in order to blunt the blood sugar increase from the carbohydrates, but I like to keep it to a minimum. I've found that as little as a t-spoon of flax oil will blunt the blood sugar increase from various carb rich breakfasts. Along with the modified cereal breakfast I listed above, this is also the time I take my fish oil capsules for the day.

A veggie omelet with half the yolks removed and a piece of whole fruit or whole grain bread would also make a decent breakfast. On the weekends when I have time, I like some of the high fiber, high protein, low carb pancake and waffle mixes. No, they're not as tasty as the real thing, but they're not a bad substitute.

However, don't let the fact that it's breakfast stop you from using your imagination. Any combination that makes a good meal any other time of the day can also be a good breakfast. Likewise, an omelet is probably a better dinner than it is a breakfast. Part of your journey to lifelong fitness is a mental one. Open up your mind to the options.

Studies repeatedly show that people who eat breakfast tend to have lower body fat than those that skip breakfast. This is the time when your body can really use the nutrients, not at night before you go to sleep. I know it may sound backwards, but people who eat a good breakfast, end up snacking less at night (when your body doesn't need the fuel). For those of you who just can't get in the habit of a real breakfast, even a piece of fruit is better than nothing.

The Rest of the Day

As a general rule of thumb, it's not a bad idea to taper the carbs as the day goes on. As I stated earlier, it's best to consume them when you need them. Lunch can have an even mix of protein, carbs, and healthy fats, but by dinner, you should try to avoid any carbs other than those present in any vegetables you are eating. You really need to get out of the habit of insisting every dinner needs a couple starch sources. Bread, potatoes, rice, etc. are completely unnecessary once your daily tasks are finished.

If weight loss is your goal, you should try to avoid snacking at all after dinner. This is absolutely the WORST time to give your body fuel. This is the also the time most people eat the worst snack food: chips, cookies, etc. are not only processed crap that is unhealthy at any time of day, but the massive quantity of carbohydrates does nothing but sit around in your blood until your body converts it to fat. Which it has plenty of time to do, since you aren't going to use them while you sleep.

If you just can't go from dinner until breakfast without something in your stomach, or if your goals are more toward building muscle or sports performance, you may want to incorporate some protein and healthy fats into an evening snack. The protein is to keep your body from eating away at your precious muscle while you sleep, with a little fat to slow the digestion. Some of my favorite choices for evening snack are sliced turkey breast and cheese or an omelet with half the yolks removed. Just be careful with quantities. You still have to plan your total calories for the day.

Workout Nutrition

If you're looking for another edge to "step up" your progress, or if you've been having problems with your energy level during your workouts, then read on.

What we're talking about here is special rules for eating before, during and after your workout. Not only does what you eat before your workout affect the quality of your workout, but what you eat after your workout affects how quickly you'll recover from a workout.

Pre Workout

First, let's talk about how you should eat before your workout. Everyone digests food a little differently, and each of us consume and process carbohydrates differently, so the timing for everyone is a little different. But we all need an adequate amount of carbohydrates in our system to fuel our muscles during the workout.

Remember, the reasons for the empty carbs in breads, pasta's etc, was to fuel our ancestor's muscles during a hard day plowing the field. While we no longer need those calorie dense carbohydrates for most of our sedentary lives, if you are doing strenuous workouts then that's the one time during the day when you can use that fuel.

This holds true even if you are trying to lose weight. Remember, the purpose of the resistance training is to prevent muscle loss while dieting and crank up your metabolism so that you burn even more calories for the days following the workout. If your workout suffers in intensity because your body lacked the proper fuel, then you've just "robbed Peter to pay Paul".

For cardio workouts, it's a little different. In this case, working out on an empty stomach may cause increased fat burning, which is great but to be honest, studies do not show any increased long term fat loss from doing cardio on an empty stomach.

So what does this mean for your pre-workout nutrition? Either have a piece of fruit on the way to the gym, or include some carbohydrates in the meal before your workout. Just be careful not to eat too close to your workout. Your body isn't good at digesting food while you're working out. The results of eating too close to the workout aren't pleasant.

What if you realize you're low on energy (due to having forgotten lunch for instance), right as you show up at the gym? Anything solid won't digest fast enough and will just sit like a rock in your stomach. You've all heard of Gatorade. Yes, for the most part it's just sugar water, and doesn't have any place in your normal daily routine, but it does do a great job in replenishing your body's energy levels at the same time that it rehydrates (perhaps more important than the energy it supplies). Someone really did their homework way back when. Gatorade doesn't have fructose like all other sugary drinks, so it's much easier for your body to use to fuel your muscles instead of just storing it as fat. For those of you who are attentive enough to notice that I recommended fruit for pre-workout nutrition, amazingly fruit has far less fructose than do sugary sodas, or Kool-aid.

I personally don't recommend making a habit of needing something right before your workout. I've found most people tend to get used to it. This is bad because you will become worn out fast and experience blood sugar drops if you don't bring your Gatorade. This was especially true for me at one point. I had gotten into the habit of sipping on a carb/protein drink during my workouts. If I'd go mountain biking or rollerblading, and try to go for longer than an hour or if I forgot my workout drink, I'd crash hard. My body had gotten used to using easily available carbs during my normal workouts, and had gotten inefficient at using its existing energy stores. Once I stopped sipping on the Gatorade during my normal workouts, the problem went away. My body went back to being able to efficiently retrieve energy from its available glycogen and fat.

Post Workout

When I first wrote this section for a newsletter many years ago, post workout nutrition was a topic only serious athletes really worried about. At that time I didn't really push my clients on this topic, as it was viewed as a little more complicated than most wanted to have to think about. However, now it seems it's a topic that's showing up more and more in mainstream health and fitness, so hopefully you won't rebel at the thought of preparing a special post workout shake. The studies are very clear on this: how you feed your body immediately after your workout is critical for recovery as well as performance and physique gains! [66,67,68,69]

After an intense workout, your body is in a state of destruction. It's actually tearing down the very muscle you're trying to build/maintain. Without proper post workout nutrition, it can stay in that destructive state for several hours, until you give it the fuel to start building. No, it's not just tearing down fat either, it's actually tearing down precious muscle tissue.

How do we stop this destructive phase? How do we start the rebuilding process where muscle is built, and fat is burned? The answer is "eat". Studies have found the optimum post workout meal is actually a combination of easily digested carbohydrates and proteins. Yes, the same insulin spiking sugars we avoid all day long just happen to be the perfect post-workout meal. Strangely enough, your body really does know what it's doing. While normally a blast of sugar would trigger an insulin spike that would immediately store that sugar as fat, after a workout your body knows that your muscles are where the sugar is really needed and it preferentially shuttles the newfound sugars directly to the muscles to jump-start the recovery process.

Along with the sugar, at this point your body can also make use of easily digested, high quality proteins. This makes sense of course, since that's what our muscles are made of. Studies seem to indicate about half as much protein as carbohydrate is about optimum for recovery.

WHAT to eat after your workout?

For recovery nutrition, fat is a big no-no. Just as fat slows digestion in any other meal, it will do the same here. This is exactly what we DON'T WANT. We want the fastest absorption possible, so stay away from all fats, even the good ones.

What does this mean you should do after a workout? Although each study shows a slightly different results, my recommendation is as follows: For an average man who is trying to put on muscle, consume 80 grams of carbohydrates and 40 grams of protein. If weight loss is the primary goal, I would probably reduce this to 60 grams of carbs and 40 grams of protein. For a woman who is trying to lose weight, about 40 grams of carbs and 25 grams of protein are about right.

I recommend using Gatorade for the carbs, and vanilla whey protein for the protein. For the 180lb guy, this would mean about 7.5 tbsp of powdered Gatorade and 1.75 scoops of whey protein powder. I recommend mixing this with about a liter of water to help re-hydrate after the workout as well.

This may seem like a huge amount of sugar to some of you, but that's the point, this is when your body really needs it.

I personally drink one of these drinks after ALL my workouts, including my cardio workouts. Recovery time is simply too important to me. I want to be ready for another workout as soon as possible. I don't worry that I might be consuming a little sugar. I don't want my upper body workout today to affect my mountain bike ride tomorrow, or vice-versa.

Of course, if you want to get a little more sophisticated, post workout is a great time to add some Branched Chain Amino Acids (BCAA's). These are some very essential proteins that your body can't manufacture on its own, and are critical to building and maintaining muscle. I add two grams of BCAA's to my workout shakes. Also, if you're interested in supplementing your diet with Creatine, the post workout drink is an ideal place to add some.

Creatine

No, Creatine is not a steroid! I feel like I just lost 10 IQ points writing that sentence, but I've seen that mistake made enough times that I thought I should start with that fact.

Creatine is a natural substance necessary for our muscles to function. It is found in our food, especially meat and fish, and is also manufactured by our bodies.

Depending on your diet, adding extra Creatine as a supplement will usually increase strength, reduce fatigue, and enhance recovery. It will also increase the size of the muscle to some extent.

Benefits have been shown in both power and endurance athletes.

Creatine is not a drug, and more is not better. Once your body has a certain amount stored, taking more will not help. Also, like I mentioned earlier, since you get it in your food supply, you may already be getting all you need.

But there is no way to know without trying. For most, the benefits will be mild, but measurable.

Creatine is inexpensive (you don't need to buy anything other than plain creatine from a reputable supplement company), and perfectly safe (no study has shown any health issues), so there really is no reason not to try it if your goals include strength or adding a little muscle.[70]

Chapter 16 – Eating for Specific Goals

"Healthy" Foods?

Before we get into advice for specific goals, I'd like to take a step back and examine the word "healthy." It seems like such an obvious word, and we all use it frequently when we talk about what we eat, but many times, I think we get confused as to what it really means.

The dictionary defines it as "conducive to good health." With "health" defined as "soundness of body or mind; freedom from disease or ailment." This is not very helpful.

What if someone is morbidly obese and they are successfully losing weight with a dangerously low calorie diet that consists only of prepackaged diet food high in artificial sweeteners, preservatives, and hydrogenated fats? If that individual is losing weight that could be causing serious and immediate health problems, then for them that food might be considered healthy, even though in the broad sense, these snacks are certainly not healthy.

The opposite is also true for many foods. Whole eggs and various nuts are certainly healthy for an individual who has control of their weight, but too much of either of these foods will

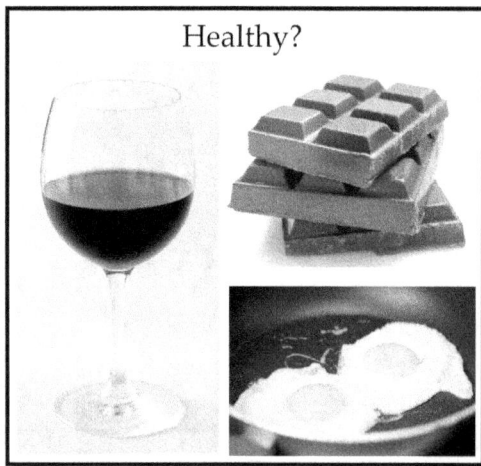

Healthy?

certainly not be conducive to weight loss and hence "health" for someone who is overweight.

How about foods like chocolate and wine? Data seems to show both of these have various healthy properties, but in excess, each has its own problems.

There's also the confusion added by changing or conflicting "expert" opinions. Eggs: how many times have they gone from healthy, to unhealthy, and back to healthy? Fish? Yes, the benefits of the omega 3 fatty acids in many fish is irrefutable, but how about mercury, or what happens when the fish are farm raised and fed a diet of corn such that their omega 3 content dwindles to next to nothing?

How about milk? Your government (primarily because of the food lobby) is always quick to point out the health benefits of a diet full of milk-based products, but in the nutrition world, milk has as many detractors as fans. Are you lactose intolerant? You may be partially and not even know it. Has the way we process milk products taken all the "good stuff" out of them? Certainly there is no longer any good fats in the milk we drink, and the protein is almost irrelevant compared to the sugar content.

Oats are a topic that really amazes me. Someone did a study that included oat bran. It was a very broad study, and the results were hardly conclusive to oat bran. But, that doesn't stop the cereal manufactures from claiming that their overly processed oat based cereal will help fight heart disease. Cheerios is even advertising the health benefits of their sugar coated cereals, even though the oats in these cereals have been processed so far beyond normal whole oats, it's hard to say if they have any real relation to whole oats. Certainly, making health claims for highly processed sugar coated oats, based on broad studies that show health benefits for raw oats is playing fast and loose with the facts.

I'm not trying to make a complete list of what is healthy and what isn't, but these two pages will at least get you thinking when you see an ad for some new overly processed "health" food.

Keep all of this in mind when choosing foods for your own personal nutrition plan. A food that may be healthy for one person's goals, may not be appropriate for another.

Weight Loss

I want to be VERY CLEAR about this! I do NOT recommend ANY special weight loss diet plans! If you define the success of a diet as not only losing the weight but also keeping it off, NONE of these short-term diets work!

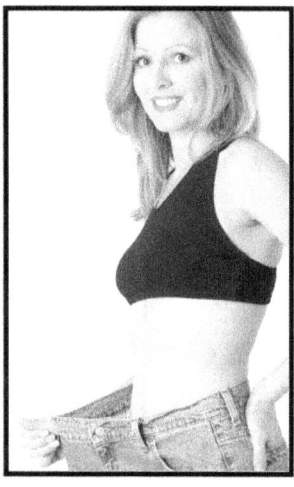

If you do not establish PERMANENT, HEALTHY, eating habits that you can maintain for the rest of your life, you WILL FAIL! Trying to tell yourself "I'll lose the weight with this crazy diet, THEN I'll learn to eat right" NEVER WORKS!

Please go back and re-read the above two paragraphs. If you do not understand and believe what I am saying here, you are destined to failure. Whether it's your workouts or how you eat, anything that you cannot maintain for the rest of your life is destined to fail. I've simply watched it too many times with too many clients.

This is the reason this section may seem a little short to some people. Most of the discussion so far is just about healthy eating in general. If you follow the above recommendations, you will probably never have to worry about your weight again. The modifications you'll want to make for the initial weight loss are just not that complicated.

First, you'll need to take the above advice VERY seriously. If you want to really start dropping body fat, you'll need to eliminate ALL simple sugars or processed carbohydrates as well as all bad fats. This means no pasta, bread, potatoes, or any fried foods. If your goals are serious, this shouldn't be a problem.

Keep protein intake the same, and get enough good fats, especially omega-3's. I still recommend supplementing with fish oil capsules even when you're trying to lose body fat. This extra healthy fat will not hurt your goals.

It always helps to plan all of your meals if possible. At the very least, plan-out some healthy, low carb snacks as part of your daily calorie intake. You know you're going to get hungry at some point and the last thing you want to do is have the snack machine at work as your only alternative.

At the start of your fat loss plan, you should keep a detailed food log as we discussed previously. Not only will this allow you to properly refine your eating habits, but it will also make you accountable. Most people don't realize just how much they're eating until they keep a food log. This is no small deal. The success rate I've seen with people who keep an honest food log is easily twice the success rate for those who don't

Don't try to lose more than a pound or two a week. Any more than that and most of your weight loss will be muscle.

There are many issues we all struggle with when we're trying to lose weight. While technically it is as simple as it sounds to lose weight, we all know that in the real world it's just not that easy. Some issues, like a craving for cheesecake (the WHOLE cheesecake), MUST be dealt with by exerting self-control. There really is no substitute for a certain amount of self-control when it comes to any sort of real change in your life. Whether it's losing weight, quitting smoking, abstaining from alcohol or gambling, there may be many tricks to help you change, but it really does come down to self control at some level. Anyone who tells you otherwise is trying to sell you something (and not something useful either)!

Weight Loss Tricks

However, there are tricks to make it easier. If you don't have to put up with small portion sizes, constant hunger pangs, and boring food, it gets A LOT easier. Not all of the following tips will sound appealing to everyone, but hopefully, you can pick up one here and there to help with the difficulties that go with losing weight.

For the most part these tips involve diluting your diet with low calorie "filler" foods. If you do any research, you'll find more studies than you might imagine that show that people who eat more fruits and vegetables tend to have less body fat than those that don't. Although fruits and vegetables do contain nutrients that our bodies need, I don't think it's quite that sophisticated. My guess is that people who eat their veggies weigh less simply because these food sources are simply less "calorie dense" than the man made alternatives.

Here are some specific hints for weight loss:

- Add some sort of protein to every meal. Protein not only slows digestion, making you feel full sooner, but it also will cause you to feel full for longer. This is the opposite of refined carbohydrates, which are absorbed quickly, and will cause you to be hungry soon thereafter.
- Eat solid meals. Yes, I know, protein shakes are a great, easy, controllable meal, but solid food is absorbed slower, and will keep you full for longer. So if you are one of these people who feel hungry soon after a protein shake, you may want to switch to solid food.
- Try to avoid bland food. Remember, this is not a temporary diet. You may be temporarily eating less than you will once you've met your weight loss goals, but in order to not rebound right back to your old bad habits (and weight), you need to establish good eating habits NOW. You don't want to eat bland food forever, so you have to start to learn how to eat and prepare food that you will be happy eating for the rest of your life. Just as you experiment with non-healthy food to find recipes or restaurants that you like, so must you do the same now with healthy food.
- Presentation is key. A plain broiled chicken breast with plain broccoli not only doesn't taste very good, but just looks unappetizing. Get creative with your cooking. If you cook your meals ahead of time and store them in individual containers for the next couple of days, it really isn't that much

more trouble to cook interesting yet still low cal meals. Try low cal marinades, spices (always low-cal), cooking spray instead of sauces, butter, etc.

- Vary your meals. Some people try to eat the same things day in and day out. You will eventually get bored with these same foods, and that's when trouble starts. Check out my web site for recipes and recipe books I recommend. Remember, we're not trying to go on a traditional "diet" where we lose some weight, then immediately gain it back once we return to our normal eating habits. Rather, we are trying to establish lifelong eating habits that will keep the fat off for good. If the food you eat is bland and repetitive, then you certainly won't stick with the program for life.

- Eat an apple BEFORE meals. This fruit is high in fiber and digests slowly, which will fill you up and cause you to want to eat less at mealtime. People who do this will actually eat less total calories, INCLUDING the calories from the apple.

- Consider lean meat alternatives to high fat protein sources. I don't feel there is anything "unhealthy" about high fat beef, pork, whole eggs, etc. (just ask the Alaskan Eskimo whose diet is VERY high in saturated fat, yet incidence of heart disease is very low), but these high fat protein sources are higher in calories than a leaner source. Which sounds more filling: a 10 oz chicken breast or a 5 oz pork chop? Or how about an omelet made from a single whole egg, or a whole cup of Egg Beater? Both have the same calories.

- Fibrous veggies are excellent filler foods for meal times (as well as being nutritious). A plate full of broccoli will fill anyone up. NO ONE gets fat on broccoli. The trick is to cook and season it so that it's consistently appetizing. Some low fat melted cheese (be careful how much) can really add to the taste factor.

- Just can't get by without some dessert before bedtime? Try sugar free gelatin with sugar free whipped topping.

- How about beverages? Non-diet soda is a real no-no! I recently did a quick calculation for a friend who said he just can't give up his non-diet soda. He was consuming 135,000 calories per year on soda. That's 45lbs per year he has to burn off. Of course, you should really consider eliminating all sugared drinks. This includes not only sodas but also fruit juice. We all know that plain water is the best beverage for your diet, but if you need something with a little flavor to persuade you to get your hydration for the day, consider lightly sweetened Ice tea, or "Propel" fitness water from Gatorade, which has only 8 calories per bottle.
- Alcoholic beverages are another area that really sabotages a lot of people's diets. I know I said earlier that you shouldn't make any changes that you can't keep up long term, but it's not a bad idea to cut back a little while you're trying to lose weight. There are some specifics later in the chapter.
- Do you really miss having a sandwich? We have become very used to eating on the run, and the sandwich is certainly a great way to carry around some meat, cheese and a few veggies. It's very hard for most of us to give up bread altogether. My solution to that is to stick with high fiber breads, and even better, high fiber rollups. Don't just grab the first loaf of "Whole Wheat" bread. Most of them are just died white bread. Take a look at the fiber content. There should be three or more grams of fiber per slice. The more, the better. I tend to look for high fiber bread that is also "light". Some of the denser whole grain, high fiber breads are really good as far as nutritional value and taste, but are so high in calories, that they aren't of much use for someone trying to lose weight. I've had good luck finding bread in regular grocery stores with 35 calories, 3 grams of fiber, and 2 grams of protein per slice.
- Many people just can't get used to the thought of dinner without some sort of potato. A good substitute for mashed potatoes is cauliflower based mashed "potatoes".

- For pasta, spaghetti squash makes an excellent and very tasty substitute for the real thing.

So there you go, some tips for making your meals a little more filling and palatable, while still being reasonably low in calories. No, it's not fried chicken, a baked potato, and an ice cream sundae for dessert, but at least it's better than a tasteless chicken breast at every meal.

If the above recommendations are not working for you, then you're doing something wrong. If you have to resort to drastic temporary diets that you will never stick with long term, you are dooming yourself to failure. The solution is probably a careful food log of everything you eat, along with an honest evaluation of what parts of my advice you are really following and what parts you are ignoring.

For many of you, this is not going to be easy, but if it were easy (and if the easy solutions offered in every other diet book really worked), then we'd all be thin and fit.

Gaining Muscle

This is a much more complicated subject than I have space to discuss. Chances are if you're seriously trying to put on large amounts of muscle then you'll probably be looking elsewhere for information that is more specialized. However, some of you may want to put on a little muscle without getting "huge" and that's what I'm focusing on here.

There are two types of people we need to discuss when it comes to trouble putting on muscle: the first is the person who has struggled with their weight, is now down to a reasonable body weight but wants to firm up.

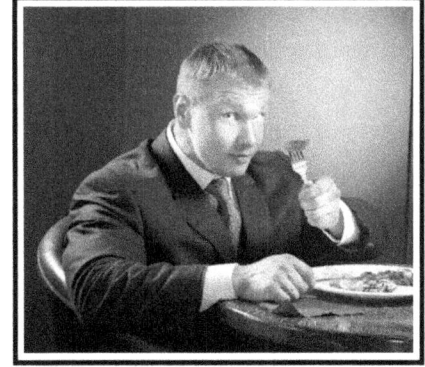

The second type is the person who has never been able to put on weight of any kind. This could be the skinny guy or the girl whose girlfriends envy her slight figure, but who wishes she had some definition in certain areas.

Muscle vs. Bodyfat

Do you remember the episode of South Park where Cartman decides to get huge and starts guzzling "Weight Gain 4000"? He thinks he's getting huge and muscular, but in reality, he's only getting huge. For many, this dilemma is very real.

The person who has a hard time putting on muscle without gaining fat is going to have some conflicting issues. For the first few months, they may put on muscle just by working out, but eventually, they'll need to worry a little more about what they are eating. For the person who has problems maintaining a low body fat level, putting on muscle without gaining body fat will be a slow struggle. This is not to say it's not possible, but just tougher.

In order to put on muscle, you must consume extra calories. Unfortunately, your body doesn't know that you just want muscle, and will try to put on fat as well. You absolutely MUST keep your diet as clean as possible. Try to eat as much quality protein and good fats as you can, and keep the carbs to only before and after your workout. For you, the after workout shake is not an option, it's a necessity. It's the one time you really need to refuel and don't be shy about it.

You'll have two options: you can either eat a little too much and not worry about gaining a little body fat, then lose the fat later, or you can take longer to put on the muscle so as to not put on any extra body fat. Personally, I've found the second method takes longer, but you'll have to experiment to find what works best for you. Just don't follow the old school method of "bulking up" by gaining as much weight as possible whether it's muscle or fat. Save that strategy for the powerlifters, and pro bodybuilder taking steroids.

Just can't put on weight?

Now, if you're the beanstalk that's never been able to put on any weight of any type, you're going to have to take a slightly different strategy: Eat, eat, and eat again. Yes, you should try to eat healthy, and certainly you'll want to get enough protein, but if you're one of those types, you may have to resort to adding some ice cream and/or peanut butter to your protein shakes, and keep some high calorie (and tasty) protein bars around for those times you "forget to eat" a real meal.

This will probably be as uncomfortable for you as losing weight is for the rest of us. You really don't have much choice. You either eat and grow or don't eat and don't grow.

It won't be as difficult for the girls looking to put on a little definition as it is for the guys trying to put on some muscle all over, but the point is the same: eat.

This is more of a psychological issue than a physiological one. What I mean by that is that as I've said earlier, very few people really have fast metabolisms. Most people who are "naturally thin" really just don't like to eat much. For many women, the idea of forcing themselves to eat more will be a VERY tough challenge. What you need to remember is that if you've always been thin, any excess fat you put on as you gain muscle, will come off very quickly. Put it out of your mind for a while and just eat!

Eating for Sports Performance

Eating for sports performance is an even more complicated topic than for building large amounts of muscle, and therefore I'm only going to scratch the surface of this for amateur athletes in general. If you are even at the level of a serious amateur athlete, I highly recommend you seek out the aide of someone who specializes in your sport.

However, there are certainly some things to keep in mind for those of you who just want to play a better game of tennis, or make a few extra runs down the ski slope.

First, remember when we talked about carbs and how modern man just doesn't need them like our ancestors did? Well this is one time when that may not hold true. As with your gym workouts, your time on the field or court need fuel as well. This is especially significant if you are trying to lose weight at the same time you are participating in a sport. If you are not properly fueled your performance will not only suffer, but you might actually lose less weight overall, as you will play longer and harder if you are properly fueled.

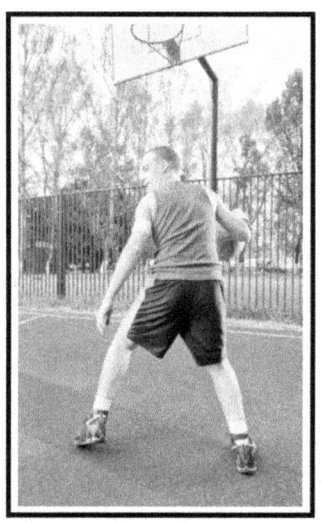

You will need to pay attention to the timing of your carbs around your workouts as discussed previously. Some pre-workout carbs, and a post workout shake will be particularly helpful if the sport consists of a lot of high intensity activity. If you're trying to lose weight as well, make sure those are the ONLY non-vegitable carbs you're eating throughout the day.

If you're really trying to improve and are playing a lot, I would love to say not to worry too much about how much you're eating, however it seems to be pretty easy for many people to out eat their sport. I've met quite a few chubby marathon runners over the years.

Just because you're running, biking, etc. does not mean you can get away with eating junk either. I know we've all seen the professional athlete who eats fast food all the time, but that's them, not us. If you want to optimize both your physique and your sports performance, you need to eat clean as often as possible.

It's unfortunate that I cannot give you a lot of specific advice. So much of that would be based on your specific needs, and the requirements of your sport as well as how often you play and any other activities you engage in. It is certainly wise to take advise from those who are competitive in your sport, but don't take their advice as gospel. Use it as a starting point and go from there. If something doesn't seem to be working: you don't have enough energy, or you're not losing the weight you want to lose, even though you're extremely active, don't just give up and think you're the exception. Keep modifying your diet until you find something that works for you.

Chapter 17 – Misc. Nutrition Topics

Supplements

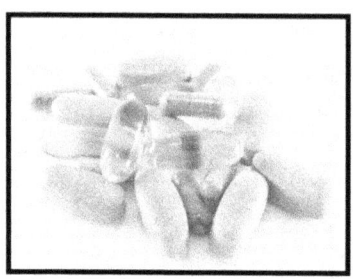

I'm not as big on supplements as many health and fitness gurus are. Back to the whole honesty thing again, as I just don't ever plan on selling anything I don't believe in. There are not many supplements I believe in. The supplements I do believe in are usually not big factors. Some may help to a small degree, but any of the goals I talk about in this book, can all be accomplished with food alone.

For the most part, I believe in whole foods. When you put a healthy food through whatever process you need to go through to get it in a bottle and get it to last (preservatives), you are usually neutralizing anything that made it good for you in the first place.

A good example of this is fiber. As simple as fiber is, it's critical for the overall nutritional value of many fruits and vegetables. Without the fiber to slow digestion, many fruits turn into sugar water when turned into liquid form. In addition, much of the nutrient content is often found in the very part of the fruit or vegetable that is taken out when it is turned into a processed supplement.

A classic example of this is apple and orange juice. Both apples and to a lesser extent, oranges can be a great part of a healthy diet, but when they are turned into their respective juice forms, they are absolutely worthless, despite what their makers might say in the commercials

Yeah, I know, I'm probably angering readers who are currently trying to get their multi-level juice businesses off the ground, but I just call it like I see it.

Hence, I'm not going to include a huge section on supplements. Occasionally, I will put an article into my newsletter or on my web site with specifics of various supplements, as that is a better place for it considering how fast the supplement landscape changes.

Multi Vitamins

About the only supplement I recommend for everyone (other than fish oil mentioned previously) is a general multi-vitamin. This one is just a big "why not?" Since I don't know what foods you eat, I really can't say what you might be deficient in, but I bet if you're like most Americans, your diet, healthy or not, does not have the variety it should. You probably eat the same foods over and over, and there are probably a few vitamins and minerals you don't get optimum amounts of.

You don't have to get fancy or expensive with this. I've never seen any real evidence that the expensive stuff is any better than a normal multivitamin.

I wouldn't worry about one brand over another, as many are just trying to add ingredients that are of questionable value.

However, I would recommend a "gender specific" formula, especially for guys. Most generic multi-vitamins have Iron, an ingredient very necessary for women, but possibly very dangerous if taken buy guys on a daily basis, as it can build up in a mans body and become toxic at some point.

Don't worry about companies who advertise how their formula is "absorbed 50% better." This stuff is so cheap, you're better off taking twice as much than pay 10 times as much for "better absorption."

Eating Out

Ok, so you're a busy professional. You travel several days out of every week. You're constantly eating out. It's just impossible to eat healthy! Right? In order to get in shape, you'd need to quit your job.

Yeah right, that's the answer. Not! You just need to start to look at things differently. If you can walk through a grocery store without buying a bunch of chips, cookies and other crap, then you can eat out and still be healthy.

It may help to examine how most of us think about eating out. Whether it's because of how we were raised, or some other reason, most of us think of eating out as a treat. As such, when we're in a restaurant, we feel we are free to order anything on the menu, and eat as much as is brought to the table. It's like all the rules that apply at home are all of a sudden swept under the rug when we walk through a restaurant door.

So your first task is to stop thinking of eating in restaurants as an excuse to cheat. There are always healthy, low cal ways to eat out.

First is restaurant selection. If you're still chowing down on fast food on a regular basis, shame on you. I know sometimes you're on the go and don't have time for a real meal, but that's when a piece of fruit or a protein bar come in handy. If you consistently find yourself in a hurry with no options, you might want to think about planning your day a little better.

Fast Food

The nice thing is, even fast food restaurants are starting to offer better choices. There are usually a couple of low cal items at most fast food restaurants, but that's not the end of the options. Those ridiculously high calorie meals that the media loves to yell about are always including a large sugar filled soda, fries, lots of mayo or other sauce, etc. Throw most of that stuff away, and choose the diet soda and side salad (w/ low cal dressing), and the meal you end up with is not that bad.

Be careful of salad dressing. That's a good warning ANYWHERE! I've seen too many healthy, low calorie salads ruined by dressing choice. This is one of the many areas where food logging will teach you SOOO much: once you start measuring out your dressing for a while, and comparing the calories in various types of dressings, you quickly learn just how bad you can damage your progress.   If you never learn this lesson, you are doomed to making the same horrible mistake over and over, and you'll be like everyone else wondering "why can't I lose the weight??"

A cheeseburger with lettuce and tomato and no bun may or may not be low cal, depending on your calorie limits, but it's a heck of a lot better than the same burger with a big bun and smothered in ketchup and mayo.   Something as simple as making the switch from ketchup or mayo to mustard can save some frequent fast food eaters upwards of 500-1000 calories per week.

I'll often order a sub and take the ingredients, fold them in half, and eat only half of the bun. Choosing a wrap is an even better alternative, but only eating half the bun can save you 200-250 calories.

Staying away from all fried foods is another big one. Even the worst fried food restaurants are now offering grilled alternatives.

Sit Down Restaurants

So what about real restaurants? It's not as hard as you may think. First, you have to get over the fact that much of the menu is junk. If you can shop for healthy foods at home, and avoid the bad stuff, why can't you avoid it on the menu? Almost every restaurant I've been to has something that's both healthy and tasty, and it's not always on the "Heart Smart" section of the menu. Here are a few of my personal favorites:

Salmon: Most places will have some sort of non-fried fish. Salmon is very common, and is easy to cook, so it usually tastes pretty good even at chain restaurants. You need to avoid the options that are covered in sauce, but since salmon has so much flavor on its own, that's not usually difficult. I'll ask for extra vegetables instead of the rolls or potato. You can't get healthier than that!

Salad: Salads aren't as boring as they used to be. Almost any restaurant will have some sort of salad with mixed greens and non-fried chicken on top. They're usually so big that they'll fill up even the biggest appetite, yet since the lettuce is so high in fiber, the calories are reasonable. Be careful not to overdo the dressing though and watch for croutons and other extras that will quickly turn a salad into a 1200 calorie disaster!

Steak: There's nothing unhealthy about a good steak. Especially if it's not covered in sauce and you skip the baked potato. Stick with the vegetables as with the Salmon above.

Roll-ups: Out for lunch with a client at one of those chain restaurants? Just because he orders a burger and fries, doesn't mean you need to. Try a chicken, turkey, or tuna roll-up. Just watch the mayo or special sauce!

Burger: Yes, I said a hamburger! We all get stuck eating bar food now and then (like when your co-workers insist on "all you can eat hot wings"). Just skip the bun, and get a side salad instead of the fries.

These are just for starters. Use your imagination. If you've got some good suggestions, put them up on my forum.

Alcohol

Alcohol and fitness isn't a topic you see in a health and fitness book very often. If you do, it's usually only advising you to not drink at all. On several occasions, I've had people question how a fitness guru could allow his clients to consume alcohol as part of their nutrition program. While it's true that hardcore fitness models and bodybuilders will certainly abstain from alcohol consumption while pursuing the perfect body, but that's probably not you.

Some of you may not drink alcohol for your own reasons, and if so, that's great, and maybe this section doesn't apply to you, but the fact is, far more of the people I've worked with do consume alcohol than don't. Telling them to abstain would not only be an impractical piece of advice, but also possibly damaging to their overall health. Every week it seems another study comes out showing the long term benefits of MODERATE alcohol consumption.

At first, it was just red wine, mainly because that was the only alcohol they studied, but more and more, the studies seem to be showing health benefits of moderate alcohol consumption in general. Some of the reported benefits of moderate alcohol consumption are: decreased risk of: coronary heart disease, dementia, high blood pressure, Alzheimer's, diabetes, rheumatoid arthritis, etc. etc.[71]

Like many things, the key is moderation. I have certainly had more than a few clients that simply could not achieve their weight loss goals until they got their partying under control. The key is to be aware of the compromises you are making, as well as being realistic about any possible harm you are doing to your body.

To many people, this issue is a heated one. I'm not trying to persuade anyone to drink or not to drink. I would highly recommend anyone who consumes, or "binge" drinks, change their habits. What is overdrinking? I'm not sure anyone has any real conclusive evidence of that, but studies seem to show that two drinks a day is safe. Obviously, if alcohol is negatively effecting your life in any way (hangovers, negative drunken behavior, family issues), then perhaps you should look at changing this part of your life.

So that we can think a little clearer on the topic, let's review some of the "facts" of alcohol consumption.

Stress Relief: One of the most widely used justifications for alcohol consumption is stress relief. It does appear to be well documented that alcohol can cause a reduction in our response to stress, but it is also well documented that drinking for stress relief can result in alcoholism. I've never seen any conclusive studies on this, and I think it's because of the fact that, as we discussed at the beginning of the book, we are all different.

What affects a person with a highly addictive personality in one way, may affect another person completely differently.

I'm one of those people who never seems to be happy unless I have twice as much on my plate as any sane individual would want. I'm also a serious worrier (runs in the family), and really tend to take my problems home with me. For me personally, there's nothing that relaxes me quite like a beer or two with my buddies at the local pub after a stressful day. But I also have a VERY unaddictive personality. I almost never over consume, and on the rare occasions that I do, it's still a lot less than most, and I can't remember the last time I had a hangover.

However, I also know many people who use drinking as stress relief, who just add more stress to their lives by drinking. I think as long as studies fail to look at different personality types, the evidence of the effects of alcohol on stress relief will always be mixed. As with many of my points in this book: Know thy self!

Liver Function: Detoxifying your blood is only one of the essential functions your liver performs. Your liver does more for you than I will try to list here. Let's just say, destroying your liver with over consumption of alcohol or any other drug that the body needs to get rid of, is something you should avoid at all costs. A healthy liver can process or detoxify alcohol at the rate of 1/4-1/2 of one drink every hour. This means if you have 5 drinks, it is probably taking upwards of 10 hours to clear your system, and your liver is being worked the entire time.

As with any other system of the body, there is a point where "work" becomes "over work." Your liver is designed to detoxify the blood, and I have yet to see any definitive study as to what level of drinking or other drug use will actually damage the liver. My guess is that as with so many other topics in this book, it's going to be different for each individual. I think we've all known someone who drank heavily every day and lived well into old age without issue. Personally, I'm not counting on being that individual. I try to err on the side of safety. My guess is that if you frequently wake up hung over, you're probably not doing your liver any favors. Also, if you regularly take other drugs that require the liver to detoxify (over the counter pain medications being the prime example), then you need to be even more careful of how much you drink.

Hangovers: There are three primary causes of hangovers. Of course, it's best to avoid them completely, but it's still interesting to understand the cause as it may shed some light on the possible long term affects of over consuming. We've already discussed the liver, and certainly overworking the liver with any sort of binge drinking will hinder its ability to clear other toxins from your system. I imagine the length of this effect is pretty much proportional to the length of time it takes your liver to clear your system of alcohol completely.

Dehydration is one of the main causes of a hangover, and perhaps the easiest to avoid. Drink lots of water before turning in for the night to minimize this effect. Or better yet, have a glass of water between each drink. This practice will have multiple benefits, perhaps the biggest being how much it will reduce the total amount you will consume.

Another cause of hangovers is the fact that alcohol destroys Vitamin C , Vitamin B6 & the amino acids L- Cysteine, & glutathione. It uses up Vitamin B1, & Vitamin B5 and breaks down tryptophan. There is decreased absorption of: Vitamin B1, Vitamin B2, Vitamin B12, folic acid, & amino acids. Alcohol induces increased urinary loss of Zinc, Magnesium, Calcium, & Vitamin B12. Eating a good meal may not help you sober up, but it will help replace the nutrients that are lost. Many alcoholics suffer malnutrition not only from these effects but because they stop eating food to compensate for the increased calories they get from the alcohol.

Certain byproducts of alcohol can bind to some of the same receptor sites in the brain as do the feel good neurotransmitters such as dopamine and serotonin. Thus, alcohol can produce a similar sense of well being. But that feeling wears off quickly &

you have to drink more to keep it going. Repeated false activation of these receptor sites sends the brain the signal to make less of these essential neurotransmitters. As a result, natural production slows and an addiction process begins. The temporary lack of these feel good hormones the morning after drinking is most certainly one of the causes of a hangover.

I won't turn this chapter into a sermon and I know most of you already know all of the following, but I don't think this discussion would be complete without listing some of the serious consequences of misuse of alcohol:

- Women who drink even moderate amounts of alcohol while pregnant have a higher risk of giving birth to a child with Fetal Alcohol Syndrome.

- Chronic intake of alcohol is associated with brain shrinkage, cognitive defects & declines in mental performance measured by neuropsychological testing. Even occasional drinking will produce declines in these tests for up to several days after drinking.

- Do I even have to go into the dangers of drinking and driving. Don't! An average women is legally drunk after as few as 2 drinks.

- Significant alcohol consumption can lower Testosterone in males by as much as 20%. Studies show this effect to be most prominent while drinking, but can last for up to a day after consumption. Also, alcohol can increase cortisol levels. Both of these effects can cause many negative effects such as: decreased muscle, increased fat storage, and decreased libido.

The take-home message of the above lecture is simply that if you are drinking a lot of alcohol and NOT meeting your fitness goals, there are far more reasons than just the calories.

Minimizing Alcohol's Effect on Your Waistline

So let's say you've already decided you're not going to give up drinking completely in order to get in shape. How can you minimize the damage? First, of course, you should minimize the amount you consume. One way to do this is to keep a daily food log and honestly log all of your alcoholic beverages along with everything else you consume. This will quickly drive home just how much damage drinking is doing to your diet, and should help you to take it easy in the future.

If you are currently drinking a half case of beer every week, cutting back to three drinks a week will result in about a pound of fat loss every two weeks. That's without doing anything else. That's 25 pounds of fat gained or lost every year!

The next best method is to watch the types of drinks you are consuming. There are two sources of calories in alcoholic beverages: the alcohol itself always contains the same number of calories, but what else is in your glass? Sugary drinks are the worst, with some dark beers taking a close second. The difference in calories is huge. The following list shows calories for a couple drinks, all having the same alcohol content:

4 oz. Glass of wine 80-90 Calories

Rum or Whiskey and diet soda 80-90 Calories

12 oz. Light Beer 90-100 Calories

12 oz. Regular Beer 120-260 Calories

4 oz. Whiskey Sour 160 Calories

8 oz. Daiquiri 500 Calories

I will repeat again that all of the above drinks have the same amount of alcohol, and will cause the same effects. Yes, that's correct, a "Parrot Head" sipping "boat drinks" will take in almost six times the number of calories that a wine drinker will for the same alcohol consumption. Switching from a Whiskey Sour or a Gin and Tonic to a Whiskey and Diet or a Gin and Diet 7up can almost cut your calories in half.

As if that wasn't a good enough reason to watch what you drink as well as how much, I recently saw a study that backed up something I've always intuitively suspected: the calories in the alcohol itself may not count as much as normal calories. This recent study was definitely not conclusive, but it seemed that subjects who consumed alcohol in a measured calorie nutrition program did not gain as much weight as predicted. I've always

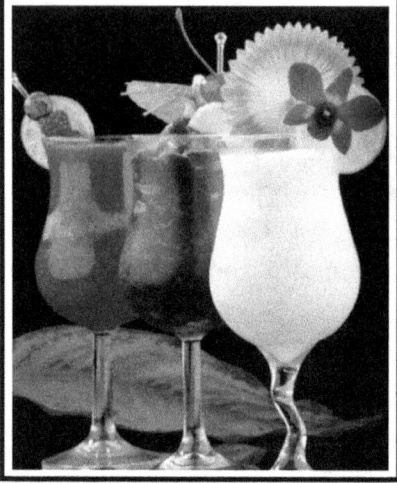

It's not the alcohol in these that will ruin your diet, it's the 1200 calories of sugar!!

noticed that as long as I'm drinking light beer, I don't notice any real effect on my body fat level. I suspect that just as with the "sugar alcohols" used to sweeten many diet products, perhaps the body doesn't utilize the calories in alcohol the same as other calories in fat, protein, or carbohydrates. Again, this is not conclusive, but it is a good reason to stick with the simpler, lower calorie drinks

Another great tip is to alternate alcoholic drinks with a glass of water or a diet soda. Some of us have a problem being in a social setting without doing something with our hands. Some people smoke, others hang out at the hors d'oeuvres table (also not good for your diet), while many just have to have a drink in their hands. Alternating with a non-alcoholic beverage with zero calories is a great way to trick yourself.

Another factor to watch out for is the effect your drinking habits may have on your workouts. We discussed elsewhere just how important intensity and concentration are in the gym. The difference between a truly hard workout and one where you are just going through the motions is huge! I've noticed that my workouts will suffer significantly the day after I drink as few as four drinks. Certainly, for athletes of any level, this factor cannot be underestimated.

Again, this article isn't an endorsement of alcohol consumption. I think most of us can agree that many people would be better off with far less alcohol in their lives. Instead, this is intended as a "heads-up" to what you're really doing to your diet when you head to the bar.

Appendices

Appendices:

Gym Etiquette

1. Unload the bar and properly rack your weights – This one should be obvious, but judging by pretty much every gym I've ever been to, it's not as obvious as it should be. Chances are, the racks at your gym have labels that tell you which dumbbells and plates go where. Even if they are not labeled, common sense should tell you not to put a 45lb plate on top of a stack of 10lb plates. I recently was in a gym where it was nearly impossible to find a pair of dumbbells of any specific weight. They were strewn all over the gym. Seriously, your mother doesn't live here to clean up your mess. Are you really that lazy that you can't put the weights back in the correct place?!

2. Don't get in the personal space of someone in the middle of a set. It doesn't take much to get injured when you're lifting heavy weights. A small bump while someone is lifting can really mess them up. Don't be lazy, find a path that doesn't lead you near them. By the same logic, if you are setting up for a set, make sure you're in an area that is appropriate: grabbing a dumbbell off the rack then standing right in front of the unused dumbbells makes it hard on everyone else to work out around you.

3. Don't hog the machines or benches. I realize many people won't take my advice to stick to fast paced workouts, but do you really need to take a nap on one of the two flat benches in the entire gym? This tends to be a problem with the machines more than the free weights, but the principle still holds true. If you're resting between sets, get up off the equipment and give someone else a chance to use it. Your momma taught you to share, didn't she?

4. Don't curl in the squat rack! Are you really that lazy that you can't pick the 40lb barbell up off the ground! If your gym is like most, there aren't that many places to do squats and related

heavy exercises that REQUIRE a rack. Often, all of them are taken up by people doing curls and other exercises that do not require a rack. This also holds true for people doing their entire routine taking up the only stretching mat in the gym, or using one of the only two flat benches in the gym to hold your bottled water!

5. No perfume or cologne. Yes, you should smell decent, but accomplish that by bathing, not by covering up the odor. People who wear too much perfume are annoying anywhere, but particularly in the gym where concentration is key. Besides, I'm working out, hence I need OXYGEN, not fumes.

6. Don't wear tight clothing unless you can REALLY pull it off. Most people can't and usually the people who can are the ones are wearing loose clothing anyway. On a similar note PLEASE wear underwear, especially if wearing loose shorts! Girls, if you are wearing a tight, skimpy outfit, expect people to stare.

7. DO NOT GIVE ADVICE! Unless someone asks you for it, do not give exercise advice no matter how bad their form is, or how much you think you know about exercise. No one will ever appreciate it. Feel free to ASK for advice, but only if it is obvious the person is resting between sets. I know, this one's tough. Once you start to learn how to work out correctly, you'll see people doing things that ABSOLUTELY WILL result in eventual injury! I've seen some of the worst heavy deadlifts with rounded lower back! It's not that I don't want to help, it's just that I know that any advice that wasn't asked for is never heeded. You'll only end up being "that guy"

9. Wipe down the equipment if you're leaving a puddle. Sweating is expected in the gym. Being too lazy to wipe it up is not.

10. Don't drop the weights. It's not good for you, or the weights. On a similar note, don't slam the weights on the stack on the machines. It's distracting to others, and bad for the equipment.

11. Keep the unnecessary noise down. A loud grunt every now and then is acceptable, but putting on a show or loud conversations to your stock broker on your cell phone really don't belong in the gym.

12. Don't try to compete with the guy or girl next to you. Lift the weight you intended to lift. Don't hurt yourself or distract him by trying to play "one up" games.

13. Use the lockers. Don't carry your gym bag around the gym. This goes for those with cell phones, magazines, multiple water bottles, etc. The gym is probably congested enough as it is. Take whatever you need for your workout and leave the rest in the locker.

14. Please be courteous in the locker room. Don't sit around naked, don't leave a mess, don't leave your lock on the locker overnight, give others some space, etc. etc.

15. This one is for Gym owners: This stuff is catching on! I know the fancy machines sell memberships, but at some point you need to start taking care of your real customers. Take a look around your gym and if there is frequently a line for the dumbbells and free weight benches, maybe it's time you sold some of those silly machines and added more free weights!

So you want to be a personal trainer?

Surprisingly, more often than I would expect, I get questions from clients and friends regarding starting a new career as a personal trainer. While most of them are well intentioned, many of them are very misguided.

Many of them think personal training is easy. They think all it takes is a couple of classes and they can spend their day in the gym, working out and socializing with clients. They see trainers charging $50-$100 an hour and they say to themselves: "That's more than I make!!"

While they are correct that personal training can be a very satisfying career for certain people, it is by no means as easy as it looks and usually a lot less financially lucrative than they expect.

First, you have to realize that there are very few successful personal trainers, and they have built up their schedules over years of hard work. When you first start out, you may be charging $60 per hour, but the gym you work out of is probably taking half of that, and you'll be spending most of your time prospecting, networking, or giving free sessions in order to obtain new clients (Zero $$ per hour).

Even once you have established your clientele, you'll still have to pay a cut to your gym, and there will still be a lot of your time that isn't compensated.

What about "in home" training? You're going to avoid paying half your fees to a gym by going to people's homes? Ok, what about travel time and auto expenses? I know in home trainers that easily spend half their time on the road (where they're not getting paid).

Over the years, I have employed over 100 personal trainers of all ages and backgrounds. Many of them really loved their new careers, but most of those were younger people who were more willing to put in the necessary time. By far the highest failure rate I had with employees was with already established professionals in other fields that were "burnt out" and decided they wanted to enjoy their job, even if it meant a pay cut. They never lasted more than a month.

Are you a stay at home mom, or retired, and think personal training would be something fun to do while the kids are at school or during your spare time? Well you better have kids that go to school at 5am or your spare time better be at any time other than the middle of the day. People want to train before or after work. Unless you're well established and VERY in demand, you'll pretty much be working from 5am-10am then you'll come back in to work from 3pm-8pm.

So none of this has dissuaded you, and you still want to give personal training a try? First of all, what are your qualifications? Just because you lost a lot of weight isn't a good qualification. Are you ready to put in the time and money to get the proper training? There are a ton of utterly useless personal trainers running around out there. Some of them are good at motivating their clients and selling their services, but most of them are pathetically lacking in the technical skills necessary to truly change their client's lives in a positive way.

There are many certification programs out there that range from completely worthless, to a pretty decent start, but none of them actually give you the training on how to train. Check out my web site for some recommendations, but if you really plan to hit the ground running, you'll need to get more than a certification. There are several schools out there that will train you how to train. One of the best in my opinion (as of the writing of this book) is National Personal Training Institute. It's a very intensive six month program.

Further Information

Did this book whet your appetite for knowledge? Are you interested in more information about health and fitness so that you can be even more productive and efficient in your workouts and nutrition? Go to my web site (www.thinkingpersonsfitness.com) for a list of other books I recommend.

Do you want more advice from me? Post a question on my online forum. I try to answer as many as I can.

Although I no longer run a chain of personal training studios, my passion for fitness and the joy I get from helping those who truly want to help themselves is still there. Today, I find I can serve more people by writing articles and books, lecturing, etc.

I will occasionally do personal fitness "makeovers" for those who have really decided it's time for a change, and I'll also do small seminars, with 4 to 6 people per seminar. If you'd like more information, contact me through my web site.

References:

General:

i - Baechle, Earl (2008) Essentials of Strength Training and Conditioning, 3rd edition, National Strength and Conditioning Association.

ii - Tesch, P. (1999) Target Bodybuilding. Champaign, IL. Human Kinetics

iii - McGill, S. (2002) Low Back Disorders. Human Kinetics

iv - McGill, S. (2004) Ultimate Back Fitness and Performance.

v - Zatsiorsky, V. (1995) Science and Practice of Strength Training. Champaign, IL. Human Kinetics

vi - Tesch, P. (1999) Target Bodybuilding. Champaign, IL. Human Kinetics

vii - Bompa, T. (1998) Serious Strength Training. Champaign, IL. Human Kinetics

viii - www.tmuscle.com various articles

Specific:

[1] US Bureau of Labor Statistics
http://www.bls.gov/news.release/atus.t01.htm

[2] NIH Publication No. 06–3680
http://win.niddk.nih.gov/publications/understanding.htm

[3] Shetty PS, Henry CJK, Black AE, et al. Energy requirements in adults: an update of basal metabolic rate (BMR) and physical activity levels (PALS). European Journal of Clinical Nutrition. 1996, 50:S11-S23.

[4] Wein, H, Stress and Disease: New Perspectives. The NIH Word On Health. October 2000
http://www.nih.gov/news/WordonHealth/oct2000/story01.htm

[5] Maxwell, B. Gastric Bypass Surgery Complications - 19 Potential Issues. http://ezinearticles.com/?expert=Blaine_Maxwell

[6] LaFalce, L. Bariatric Surgery - Expenses, Risks, and Insurance Coverage. http://EzineArticles.com/?expert=Laura_LaFalce

[7] Gordon, S. Studies Highlight Risks of Bariatric Surgery
http://news.healingwell.com/index.php?p=news1&id=528605

[8] Maggard MA, Shugarman LR, Suttorp M, et al. (2005). "Meta-analysis: surgical treatment of obesity". Ann. Intern. Med. 142 (7): 547–59.

9 Abell TL, Minocha A (2006). "Gastrointestinal complications of bariatric surgery: diagnosis and therapy". Am. J. Med. Sci. 331 (4): 214–8.

10 Malcolm K. Robinson, Editorial, Surgical treatment of obesity -- weighing the facts, N Engl J Med, 361:520, July 30, 2009

11 Mayo Clinic Staff. Gastric bypass surgery http://www.mayoclinic.com/health/gastric-bypass/MY00825

12 http://www.musclebeach.net/

13 Gutin B, Kasper MJ 1992 Can vigorous exercise play a role in osteoporosis prevention? A review. Osteop Int 2: 55-69.

14 Iwamoto J., T. Takeda S. Ichimura (2001) Effect of exercise training and detraining on bone mineral density in postmenopausal women with osteoporosis. J. Orthop.Sci. 6:128-132.

15 Kemmler, et all. Long-Term Four-Year Exercise Has A Positive Effect on Menopausal Risk Factors: the Erlangen Fitness Osteoporosis Prevention Study, Journal of Strength & Conditioning Research. 21(1):232-239, February 2007.

16 Schwanbeck, S, Chilibeck, PD, and Binsted, G. A comparison of free weight squat to smith machine squat using electromyography. J Strength Cond Res 23(9): 2588-2591, 2009.

17 Mehdi. Smith Machine: 10 Reasons Why You Shouldn't Use It for Squats. http://stronglifts.com/smith-machine-squats-power-rack-free-weights/

18 Cooper, K. (2005) Regaining the Power of Youth. Thomas Nelson

19 Myers J, Prakash M, Froelicher V, et al. Exercise capacity and mortality among men referred for exercise testing. N Engl J Med. 2002; 346: 793–801.

20 Treuth, M.S., Hunter, G.R., & Williams, M. (1996). Effects of exercise intensity on 24-h energy expenditure and substrate oxidation. Medicine and Science in Sports & Exercise, 28, 1138-1143

21 King, J., Panton, L., Broeder, C., Browder, K., Quindry, J., & Rhea, L. (2001). A comparison of high intensity vs. low intensity exercise on body composition in overweight women. Medicine and Science in Sports & Exercise, 33, A2421

22 Pichot, V. Interval training in elderly men increases both heart rate variability and baroreflex activity. Springer. Apr 2005

[23] Earnest, C. The role of exercise interval training in treating cardiovascular disease risk factors. Current Cardiovascular Risk Reports. Springer. Jan 2009.

[24] McGill, S. (2002) Low Back Disorders. Human Kinetics 118-120

[25] FRY, ANDREW C.; Smith, J. Chadwick; SCHILLING, BRIAN K. Effect of Knee Position on Hip and Knee Torques During the Barbell Squat. Journal of Strength & Conditioning Research. November 2003 - Volume 17 - Issue 4

[26] Contreras, B. Inside the Muscles: Best Chest and Triceps Exercises. www.tmuscle.com

[27] NeLM. Do Non-Steroidal Anti-Inflammatory Drugs affect fracture healing post-operatively? September 2006. http://www.druginfozone.nhs.uk/Record%20Viewing/viewRecord.as px?id=570359

[28] Vuolteenaho K, Moilanen T and Moilanen E. Non-steroidal anti-inflammatory drugs, cyclooxygenase-2 and the bone healing process. Basic Clin Pharmacol Toxicol. 2008 Jan;102(1):10-4. http://www.hubmed.org/display.cgi?uids=17973900

[29] Paoloni JA et al. The use of therapeutic medications for soft-tissue injuries in sports medicine. MJA 2005; 183 (7): 384-388 http://www.mja.com.au/public/issues/183_07_031005/pao10246_fm.h tml

[30] Cholewicki, J., and McGill, S.M. (1992) Lumbar posterior ligament involvement during extremely heavy lifts estimated from fluoroscopic measurements. Journal of Biomechanics, 25(1):17.

[31] Nutter,P. (1988) Aerobic exercise in the treatment and prevention of low back pain. State of the Are Review of Occupational Medicine, 3: 137.

[32] McGill, S. (2002) Low Back Disorders. Human Kinetics, 12

[33] McGill, S. (2002) Low Back Disorders. Human Kinetics, 127

[34] FRY, ANDREW C.; Smith, J. Chadwick; SCHILLING, BRIAN K., Effect of Knee Position on Hip and Knee Torques During the Barbell Squat, The Journal of Strength & Conditioning Research. November 2003 - Volume 17 - Issue 4

[35] McGill, S. (2002) Low Back Disorders. Human Kinetics, 12

[36] Baechle, Earl (2008) Essentials of Strength Training and Conditioning, 3rd edition, National Strength and Conditioning Association. 300-301

[37] Center for Disease Control. www.cdc.gov/obesity

[38] Agel, J, Arendt, EA, and Bershadsky, B. Anterior cruciate ligament injury in national collegiate athletic association basketball and soccer: a 13-year review. Am J Sports Med 33: 524-530, 2005.

[39] Malina,R. Physical activity and training: Effects on stature and adolescent growth spurt. Med Sci Sports Exerc 26:759-766. 1994

[40] Vicente-Rodriguez. How does exercise affect bone development during growth? Sports Med 36:561-569. 2006

[41] Faigenbaum. Strength training for children and adolescents. Clin Sports Med 19:593-619. 2000

[42] Kraemer,W.,A.Fry,P.Frykman,B.Conroy,J.Hoffman. Resistance training and youth. Pediatr Exer Sci 1:336-350. 1989

[43] Faigenbaum,A.L.Zaichkowsy,W.Wescott, L.Micheli, A.Fehlandt. The effects of a twice per week strength training program on Children. Pediartr Exerc Sci 5:339-346. 1993

[44] American Academy of Pediatrics. www.aap.org

[45] American Academy of Family Physicians. www.aafp.org

[46] Baechle, Earl (2008) Essentials of Strength Training and Conditioning, 3rd edition, National Strength and Conditioning Association. 142-153

[47] Krieger, J., Sitren, H., Daniels, M., Langkamp-Henken, B. (2006). Effects of variation in protein and carbohydrate intake on body mass and composition during energy restriction: a meta-regression 1. *The American Journal of Clinical Nutrition, 83*(2), 1442-1443.

[48] Frestedt, J., Zenk, J., Kuskowski, M., Ward, L., Bastian, E. A whey-protein supplement increases fat loss and spares lean muscle in obese subjects: a randomized human clinical study. Nutr Metab (Lond). 2008; 5: 8

[49] Layman DK, Boileau RA, Erickson DJ, Painter JE, Shiue H, Sather C, Christou DD. A reduced ratio of dietary carbohydrate to protein improves body composition and blood lipid profiles during weight loss in adult women. J Nutr. 2003;133:411–417

[50] Tarnopolsky, MA; Atkinson, SA; MacDougall, JD; et al. Evaluation of protein requirements for trained strength athletes. J Appl Physiol. 1992 Nov;73(5):1986-95.

[51] Poortmans, JR and Dellalieux, O. Do regular high protein diets have potential health risks on kidney function in athletes? Int J Sport Nutr Exerc Metab. 10(1), 28-38, 2000

[52] LaBounty, P, et al. (2005). Blood markers of kidney function and dietary protein intake of resistance trained males. J Int Soc Sports Nutr.2:5.

[53] Critser. (2003) Fat Land, How Americans Became the Fattest People in The World.

[54] Council on Foods and Nutrition. A critique of low-carbohydrate ketogenic weight reducing

regimes. JAMA (1973) 224: 1415-1419.

[55] Grande F. Energy balance and body composition: a critical study of three recent publications.

Ann Int Med (1968) 68: 467-480.

[56] Werner SC Comparison between weight reduction on a high calorie, high fat diet and on a

isocaloric regimen high in carbohydrate. New Engl J Med (1955) 252: 604-612.

[57] Olsson KE and Saltin B. Variations in total body water with muscle glycogen changes in man.

Acta Physiol Scand (1970) 80: 11-18.

[58] Esposito, K. et. al. Postmeal glucose peaks at home associate with carotid intima-media thickness in type 2 diabetes J Clin Endo doi:10.1210/jc.2007-2000

[59] Bardini, G. et al. Inflammation markers and metabolic characteristics of subjects with one-hour plasma glucose levels.   Diabetes Care Published online before print November 16, 2009, doi: 10.2337/dc09-134

[60] Khaw,K., Wareham,N., Bingham,S., Luben,R., Welch,A., Day,N. Association of Hemoglobin A1c with Cardiovascular Disease and Mortality in Adults: The European Prospective Investigation into Cancer in Norfolk.   Annals of Internal Medicine, 9/21/2004, Vol 141, no 6, 413-420

[61] Dr Esther van 't Riet, Elevated HbA1c Associated With Nonfatal CVD, Even in Nondiabetics. European Association for the Study of Diabetes 2007 Meeting.

[62]   http://diabetes.webmd.com/news/20040920/death-risk-rises-with-blood-sugar

[63] Zamora, A., Carbohydrates - Chemical Structure
http://scientificpsychic.com/fitness/carbohydrates.html

[64] Knopp RH, Retzlaff BM (November 2004). "Saturated fat prevents coronary artery disease? An American paradox". The American Journal of Clinical Nutrition 80 (5): 1102–3

[65] Siri-Tarino PW, Sun Q, Hu FB, Krauss RM (March 2010). "Meta-analysis of prospective cohort studies evaluating the association of saturated fat with cardiovascular disease". The American Journal of Clinical Nutrition 91 (3): 535–46

[66] Tipton et al. (2001). Timing of amino acid-carbohydrate ingestion alters anabolic response of muscle to resistance exercise. Am.J.Physiol Endocrinol.Metab. 281: 197-206.

[67] Ivy et al. (2002) Early postexercise muscle glycogen recovery is enhanced with a carbohydrate-protein supplement. J Appl Physiol. Oct;93(4):1337-44.

[68] Levenhagen et al. (2001). Postexercise nutrient intake timing in humans is critical to recovery of leg glucose and protein homeostasis. Am.J.Physiol Endocrinol.Metab. 280(6): 982-993.

[69] Van Loon et al. (2000a). Maximizing postexercise muscle glycogen synthesis: carbohydrate supplementation and the application of amino acid or protein hydrolysate mixtures. Am J Clin Nutrition. 72(1): 106-111.

[70] Baechle, Earl (2008) Essentials of Strength Training and Conditioning, 3rd edition, National Strength and Conditioning Association.

[71] Hanson, D. www2.potsdam.edu/hansondj/alcoholandhealth.html

www.ingramcontent.com/pod-product-compliance
Lightning Source LLC
Chambersburg PA
CBHW062127280526
45788CB00001B/86